MANAGING THE GIFT™
OF
YOUR ADD/HD CHILD

MANAGING THE GIFT™
OF
YOUR ADD/HD CHILD

Dr. Kevin Ross Emery

ACKNOWLEDGEMENTS

For me there is no such thing as a creative project that happens in isolation. I reach out (and sometimes drag in) people to be my sounding boards, my supporters and sometimes even my nemesis, as they keep me becoming the best me that I can be. For this book the cast of characters included:

To my niece Janis Marilyn Emery Bromfield, who through her editing assistance, got into her uncle's head, more than she ever wanted to.

Elmer J. Howard, my right hand man, who regularly switched hats from cheerleader and supporter to nemesis.

Kim Kozak, who win lose or draw in our sometimes heated discussions never failed to show up when asked.

Donna Bass, whose passion for the subject at times rivaled, if not surpassed mine.

Anita McCormick, who always kept an eye out for anything ADD/HD that might help me with the book or the blogs and sent me more then I could have ever used.

DEDICATION

To Katie Lyon-Pingree,

If I ever had a doubt about your dedication to me and this message it would have been totally erased the day you asked me the simple question, "Do you want this to be a good book or a great one?"

Upon answering, a great one, it was with and because of your time, talents, energy and love that this great book now exists. It COULD NOT have happened without your thoughtful questions, stubborn persistence and refusal to settle. Thank-you.

TABLE OF CONTENTS

Introduction xiii

Chapter 1: Review. 1

    Understanding How ADD Got Here 1

    Verbiage Clarity 5

    Physical Energy Flow Patterns 6

        Steady 6

        Pulse 7

        Crescendo 7

    Emotional Patterns 7

    Emotional Drops 7

        Hold-Drop 8

        Squeeze, Hold-Drop 8

        Hold-Drop with After-Shock 8

    Emotional Coffee Breaks 9

    Intellectual Patterns 12

        Spaghetti 12

        Pulse/Burst 12

        DSL 13

    The Spiritual Body: The ADD/HD Impact 13

    The Spiritual Body: Managing the Gift .15

    Pros and Cons 18

Chapter 2: Parenting. 21

The Evolving Parent 21

Shifting Behaviors. 23

    Emotionally Based Approach. 23

    Assigning Value Approach. 24

Over-Praising 25

Actions and Consequences. 25

Battles of the Wills. 27

Increasing Focus Through Diet 27

Play 29

Body and Energy Awareness 30

Unwilling Willing Disobedience. 31

Advocate. 32

Chapter 3: Side Effects of Being ADD/HD in a Non-ADD World. . . 35

    Low Self-Esteem 35

    Low Self-Worth. 37

    Depression 38

    Stubbornness and Resistance to Change 40

    Anxiety. 43

    Isolation 43

    Shame and Guilt. 44

    Fear. 45

Challenges of Language. 47

Helping Your Child with Anxiety, Isolation, Shame and Fear. 49

Chapter 4: Learning 51

Hooked on Learning 51

Assignment of Value 51

Mindless Memorization. 53

Curiosity. 53

Imagination 54

Helping Your Child Learn by "Painting Their Portrait" 54

What Is Their Canvas 55

Learning Styles 56

    Auditory Learning. 56

Visual Learning. 56

Kinesthetic Learning. 57

Processing Styles 58

External 58

Internal. 59

Recharging Styles 60

Thinking Styles. 60

Analytical 61

Abstract 61

Spiral 61

Information Handling. 63

Creating The Portrait 64

Your Child's Style 64

ADD/HD Intellectual Patterns 65

ADD/HD Energy Patterns. 65

Thought, Attachment, and Processing Styles 66

Chapter 5: Supporting and Guiding 69

Transitions 70

Introverted-Internal. 71

Extroverted-Internal 73

Extroverted-External 73

Introverted-External 74

Out in the World 75

Helping Them Fly. 76

Strategies 79

Chapter 6: Teaching 83

Inventive Ways to Teach ADD/HD Child 83

Proof of Proficiency Learning. 85

Doer. 88

Teacher. 88

Facilitator 88

Innovator 89

Chapter 7: Taking a Closer Look at the DSM-IV 91

Genetics 93

Inattention 93

Hyperactivity/Impulsivity 95

General Criteria 96

Mental Status Examination 98

Environment 100

Chapter 8: Medications, Manipulation, Money and Musings 101

Managing the Gift 101

Everybody is Making Money on ADHD, But at What Cost? 103

Why All the Focus on Medications? 104

For Whose Benefit Do We Drug Our Children? 107

FDA Approved Drugs 109

The ADHD Scam and the Mass Drugging of School Children 112

Drugging the Children in America: 84% of ADHD Kids Put on
Medication 114

The Business of ADHD. 117

Chapter 9: Supporting Cast 121

Chiropractic 123

Homeopathy 124

Flower Essences 125

Biofeedback/ Neurofeedback 125

Ingestions: Supportive and Otherwise 127

Heroes and Villians 127

Sidekicks 129

Therapeutic Magnets 130

Full Spectrum Lighting 131

Cleansing and Detoxing 131

Energy Work. 132

To Keep in Mind. 133

Chapter 10: In Conclusion 135

INTRODUCTION

TIMING IS EVERYTHING. Because of the time I was born in and the parents that I had, I completely dodged both being medicated for ADD/HD and the label that goes with it. That probably had something to do with the fact neither had yet been created. But I was not alone in dodging that bullet, but rather I was in very good company. A plethora of the architects of the twentieth century dodged it as well, but we will stay focused on me for the moment since we know focus is one of the issues after all.

When I was in kindergarten my parents were called and asked to come in because I was struggling in school. Papa insisted that I be included in the meeting. They resisted the idea but he wouldn't relent. Once we got there they told my parents that they felt that it would be best if I were put in the slow class. That although I was enthusiastic and a joy to be around, I obviously couldn't keep up and it would be better for me. With some extra help I might be able to be moved back into a class with my peers at some point. My mother, who was not good at challenging authority figures, was ready to acquiesce. However Papa, the trouble maker (and who I take after) was not as quick to agree. Through asking probing questions what he learned was that every time the teacher asked a question I would end up getting really excited, jump up and down and raising my hand. When the teacher called on me I would then either fumble through a very confusing answer or struggle to get out anything at all. So Papa asked me to come sit on his knee, he wrapped his arm around me and held me to him and then told the teacher to ask one of the questions.

The teacher asked and I got all excited because I knew the answer but before I could speak my father instructed me to take a deep breath and think about what I needed to say and then say it. By doing that I got the answer right and got the right answer to every other question that they could think to ask me that day. By the time we finished, Papa told them that maybe I did need to be in another class but not the slow class however I needed to be in a class where a teacher knew how to work with a very bright child.

If I had been born ten years later I might have been put in a class for gifted children, and Papa would have loved that. Because I was bright, restless, got bored easily, asked too many questions and had too much energy.

If I had been born fifteen years later they would have tried to label me ADD and medicated me just because I was bright, restless, got bored easily, asked too many questions and had too much energy. Papa would have never allowed that.

When I wrote my first book on ADD: Managing The Gift™: *Alternative Approaches To Attention Deficit Disorder*, I had no concept that I, myself would ever be considered ADD. As Papa always said, "There are none so blind as those who choose not to see". When people asked me if I was ADD I would just laugh. By that point I figured out that I had had significant others who were, plenty of clients and even some friends, but not me. Why? Because I saw the ADD individual as one who was wildly creative, very brilliant and looked at the world from a whole different perspective, high energy and very intense when focused on something. My closest friends, students and life partner would say "…and so your not ADD, why?", when I gave them the criteria, because I am not bright enough, or creative enough or I don't think outside of the box enough, they would shake their heads and walk away. I finally got it. I also finally got how deeply impacted I had been in my own childhood by not fitting in, by being told I was stupid or would never make anything of myself (after my mother and father divorced and he became a lesser force in my upbringing).

Through helping children and adults with ADD/HD over the last dozen years or so help them discover their own gifts, helping them embrace their self-worth and develop a healthier self-esteem, I found mine in places where I didn't even know those things were missing. Mostly because they had become very subtly interwoven in ways that kept them hidden from me._

And so because I am ADD/HD, I hyper focused on understanding and figuring how to explain, help and work with ADD/HD and then went on to other things. A dozen years ago ADD/HD, as an issue, kidnapped me and my practice. I became completely emerged in it, developing protocols, teaching workshops, doing in-services, writing articles and finally making it the core of my doctoral program with my thesis on the subject becoming my first book. Then at some point, I burned out, focused my energies and practice on other issues, helping people in other ways. Now, I have been called back.Many things I said ten years ago, in the first book, are beginning to be recognized as valid. The alarmingly increasing rate of children being diagnosed, and medicated, that I predicted so long ago, has also come to pass and the school system that I said was failing not just our ADD/HD children but all children is finally falling apart enough that we may finally have the courage to tear it down and build a system that will work.

I never stopped working altogether with individuals gifted with ADD/HD, they just have not always been my focus. Along the way came the idea of the Managing The Gift ™ series. This book, *Managing The Gift*™ *Of your ADD/HD Child* felt like the right place to begin. As time goes on you can look for *Managing The Gift*™ *of the ADD/HD Entrepreneur* & *Managing The Gift*™ *of Your ADD/HD Life Partner* and I wouldn't be surprised if there were others but these will start. But always first will be *Managing The Gift*™: *Alternative Approaches For Attention Deficit Disorder.*

I will begin this book with a basic review of the first one to make sure, as one of my old bosses used to say, we are singing off the same piece of music. Than we shall cover four basic areas of working with your child; parenting, teaching, supporting and guiding. I will introduce concepts and ideas that have evolved through my last decade of work and continued discovery. I will use real examples and give you tools and techniques to help you help your child. Then we will move into what you need as a parent to be the bridge between your child, your child's world, and the world your child must live in. Also I have shared some other people's thoughts and perspectives in the form of blogs that I came across in the process of doing this work that I felt would be helpful. And then no book like this would be complete without some closing thoughts.

One of the challenges in creating this book was the pronoun usage in referring to the ADD/HD child. Due to the assumption that more male children then females have ADD/HD, it was suggested that I should just use the male pronoun throughout the book. However, because I disagreed with that assumption, I have chosen to alternate pronouns from chapter to chapter. Though it is true, more ADD/HD labels are assigned to male children, it is a misnomer that there are not as many female children (and adults) who are gifted with ADD/HD. It is just due to a variety of factors such as learning styles, learning and processing styles, the environmental differences in raising male children versus female children that boys are more likely to be diagnosed.

Before we go much further, I want to put a few things front and center about this book, about my work, and my view on ADD/HD. That will let you know whether this is the right book for you or not.

- I see this as an evolutionary process and as such we need to allow it to adjust the environment and work with it, not medicate it.

- The goal of that process is to broaden the bandwidth of humanity, not to replace non-ADD/HD people with ADD/HD but to "ADD" to them.

- ADD/HD people over the last century have been creating a more ADD/HD friendly and challenging environment with innovations such as computers, the internet and video games.

- ADD/HD individuals are not broken, not disabled, do not need to be fixed and are mostly handicapped by a series of choices that oftentimes they don't know or understand why they are making.

- There is a need to separate what is really an ADD/HD issue and what is an issue of the ADD/HD person living in a non- ADD/HD.

- Accept that many of our long standing institutions, including public education, are more interested in self-preservation than making the core necessary changes to serve this population.

- There is still a resistance to working with the "whole person", creating whole life solutions, adjusting thought processes and making substantive changes when necessary. Quick fixes that are symptom oriented still seem be the rule of the day.

- We want to opt out of the solutions that may fix the problems but are out of our comfort zones or even our belief systems. It's easier to give our power to the authority figures and pass our responsibilities on, when feeling overwhelmed.

- Medication is a drug'em up, dumb'em down answer.

- I do not and have not ever liked the choice of medication for these individuals as anything more that a stop gap, temporary solution or an occasional solution to one off situations.

- ADD/HD has become a billion dollar industry, and like other billion dollar industries will do what it takes to protect itself.

- It is far more convenient, and profitable to label and medicate a child then to put in the necessary time and effort to help that child blossom within their gifts, talents and uniqueness.

- Doing lots of research studies, in lots of control group settings to create lots of hypothesis are nice but common sense and practical solutions, even when not proven, win hands down with me every time.

- I am not, nor have ever pretended to be a classically trained counselor, psychotherapist or PhD. I work with very alternative methods and have a different way of seeing the world, as these kids do.

- If you are looking for a quick fix- this ain't it!

When I was commandeered into the ADD/HD arena in the late nineties, I was called everything from a half-baked kook to having the owner's manual for the ADD/HD brain. Back then, the number of children and adults who were diagnosed with ADD/HD were low, but quickly rising. The abuse factor was already beginning to kick in. There was money to be made. The organization CHADD which is the single largest provider of ADD information, was greatly funded by the drug company who produced Ritalin. All their literature pushed medication. There were a few of us lone wolves out there challenging what was going on. Some were MD's, some were PhD's, and some were just people out in the field, like me, seeing what helped and what didn't. I know of one case where an MD who came out against drugging, who had a book out, was refused to even present at the national CHADD conference. In addition, my calls to CHADD were never returned.

Over ten years ago, I identified different ways that ADD/HD impacted individuals and that it wasn't just a single impact. There were losses of brilliance, uniqueness and creativity with the uses of medication, and the list goes on. But I wasn't classically trained, I wasn't a PhD or an MD so what I said had no weight, except to those whom I helped live more successful lives without being medicated.

Only by reading some of the current popular books that have come out since mine did I now see all sorts of shades of my words coming out of some of those same PhDs' and MDs' mouths that I was discounted for over ten years ago. Well good for them, except for the fact that they continue to rush towards medication. They also continue to dismiss that the hard work of challenging the broken systems, cleaning up the atrocious eating habits and environmental toxicities still exist and would rather gravitate to the quick fix. They still see it as a disability. Some things change and some don't.

Speaking of change let's see how those ADD/HD numbers look today. These are facts taken from the Centers for Disease Control and Prevention.[1]

- As of 2007, 2.7 million youths, ages 4 to 17 years, (66.3% of those with a current diagnosis) were receiving medication treatment for the "disorder".

- In 2003, 4.3% of children with an ADHD diagnosis (2,473,000) were being medicated. By 2005, 56.3% of those children with an ADHD diagnosis were being medicated.

- Approximately 9.5% or 5.4 million children 4-17 years of age have ever been diagnosed with ADHD, as of 2007.

- The percentage of children with a parent-reported ADHD diagnosis increased by 22% between 2003 and 2007.

- Rates of ADHD diagnosis increased an average of 3% per year from 1997 to 2006 and an average of 5.5% per year from 2003 to 2007.

- Boys (13.2%) were more likely than girls (5.6%) to have ever been diagnosed with ADHD.

---

1 www.cdc.gov

- Rates of ADHD diagnosis increased at a greater rate among older teens as compared to younger children.

- The highest rates of parent-reported ADHD diagnosis were noted among children covered by Medicaid and multiracial children.

- Prevalence of parent-reported ADHD diagnosis varied substantially by state, from a low of 5.6% in Nevada to a high of 15.6% in North Carolina.

So here are some things I found interesting- after I moved past feeling angry, sad, and back into impassioned. Nineteen states are giving support to families that have labeled and medicated their children for ADHD, who are at or exceed 30% of their total SSI payout for children with disabilities, with the national average of SSI support being for families with an ADHD child hovering around 31%; in numbers around 200,000 cases. Because these "cases" can only qualify if the child is medicated the system is playing doctor/parent here. Of those 19 states, 10 are red, 7 blue and 1 is purple. Thirteen of those nineteen states are below the national household average income, including 7 out of 10 of the poorest states.

So why are the poorer, more conservative states more likely to insist on labeling and medication? Because ADD/HD children are more challenging, more rebellious, less likely to conform to the old ways of doing things always pushing forward to new and better ways of doing things. Also, they tend to be less educated, and lack availability to outside resources.

But the one fact I found most interesting that there are no monies or no support for families who are struggling financially but want to deal with their children in non-medical ways. Imagine that.

As if trying to raise an ADD/HD child is not enough to make your head spin all the AMA and drug companies' spin on the issue, political maneuvering, and lobbying agendas to the tune of hundreds of millions of dollars a year, as well as the numbers I just shared with you certainly will. So I only have one thing left to say before we begin.

Congratulations.

You have brought into your life an opportunity to grow and become more of a person you ever thought you were capable of. Being a parent to this child you are going to have to be more aware of your own thoughts, feelings, beliefs, actions. Anything that is incongruent within you this child will find and point out to you. You will not help your child learn how to be successful in the world unless you allow yourself to fully participate, understand (as best possible) and embrace their perspectives and experiences of the world around them. In that process, you not only help them better integrate into the greater world but you become a better parent and a better person in the process. Welcome to parenting an ADD/HD child.

Enjoy the journey.

CHAPTER 1

REVIEW

THERE IS NO WAY to make this a short or even quick section and still communicate what needs to be communicated. Therefore, I will be presenting information as factual that I have taken from my first book, a place where I made a case for the following suppositions. For further explanation I recommend you read the first book. If you proceed with lack of understanding or belief about those suppositions from the very beginning, then when I present the approaches and courses of action that stem from the information, they will not make sense to you. Even if you try to implement them, your issue with them will more than likely be communicated to your child, spouse or those who work with your child. Overall, it will make helping your child extremely difficult if not impossible. Also, there is information that I have included in this book that was edited out of the last book, information that had not surfaced when I did the first book, and information which I see differently ten years later. In this chapter, I am just trying to focus on what you need from the first book in order for you to get the most out of this book.

Understanding How ADD Got Here

This thing we call ADD has been around since the beginning of recorded history. Over the years as ADD shifted more and more to ADHD for any number of reasons, at least a few of them had to do with the profitability and spin that could be spun with the ADHD label over the ADD label. ADHD was easier to write prescriptions for, easier to get funding for and it played better in the media. I began using ADD/HD to make people ask me why in order to make a statement about how much we are being manipulated around this subject and the issues that get created because it is beneficial for the creator. That which today we call some version of ADD/HD is a broadening of humanities' bandwidth. In fact I would say that it is an **ADD**itional Hard **D**rive upgrade which is something that has cycled throughout history at times of great growth or great enlightenment. Humanity leaps forward with some new discovery, realization, or epiphany and then takes time to allow those changes to settle in and become accepted. Eventually the revolutionary change becomes an institution, belief system, or even status quo that permeates governments, religions and the powerful people of that particular day and age. Humanity then moves into stagnation and the established system becomes a weapon utilized by the institutions, governments and people in power to stay in power. The new becomes old and established and then the establishment looks at new ways of being or seeing something as a threat to their rule. Sooner or later every institution (governments, religions, corporations) becomes more committed to the preservation of the institution itself than to the people the institution was created to serve. Therefore, throughout history, we have these small groups of individuals that seem to topple the way things are being run either in the whole world or their particular area of the world. Often they are called rebels, troublemakers, and heretics. The earliest ones have been imprisoned, burned at stakes, and so forth. Just as often, when the ideas that they brought to the world were implemented and changed the world, they became heroes or saints. Sometimes two or three generations of them seem to show up to give us golden ages or times like the Renaissance. Aristotle, Plato, and DaVinci were people like this.

But it is different this time. This time we had some movers and shakers coming in to do a course correction for humanity that has become an evolutionary process. These individuals began coming in the 1850's and were the architects of the 20th century. They made the way for more and more children to be born with a way of seeing, thinking, and experiencing in the world which has already and will continue to leave the world a much different place than they found it.

ADD is part of an evolutionary process which has been both adjusting the environment it found and then has continued to adjust to the environment it is creating. These individuals are here to bring about change. It is a natural process of adaptation of the species. Oftentimes we think about evolution as a slow process that cannot even be identified. However, logically we must realize that small subtle changes generation after generation is exactly how evolution does happen. As certain things that no longer are required for our survival become dormant, the energies used to actively support those skill sets and ways of being are then funneled into other areas that were not crucial to our earlier existence. In other words, as we have made the physical world a safer place and our continuation of the species more solid, we now focus our expansion into other areas, such as social, emotional, intellectual and spiritual venues.

The energies we spent in hunting and gathering food shifted at some point. The focus was on raising food, whether crops or animals. When we became efficient in that process, our focus went into improving the food we were raising, and now our energies are moving into engineering food. The ADD individual is the result of a shift from we were to where we are going. Now, just as we have areas of the world and people in the world who still hunt and gather, ADD individuals are here not to replace the current version of humanity but to add to it. They bring into humanity something *ADDitional*. Perhaps the best analogy here is what happens when two different races come together. The children of that coupling have both good and bad qualities from both. As individuals who have evolved into this kind of person we now call ADD/HD couples with a non-ADD/HD person, the child will be a combination. As a result of the evolutionary process, even within a single family there might be one child who has no ADD/HD traits showing, another child who has some but not enough to be called ADD/HD and yet a third child who is ADD/HD version 2.0. This third child could be a mixture of some traits of the ADD/HD parent which were taken to the next level, some traits from the non-ADD/HD parent and then the rest of their makeup became stimulated or heightened by being exposed to a world that is becoming more and more ADD/HD in how it functions.

Originally as these children began to stand out within the classrooms, it was because of their restlessness, boredom, brilliance and acting out that we created gifted children programs for them. Then as their numbers grew, we took the same criteria and began labeling them ADD/HD and decided we no longer had the resources, time and energy for gifted children. I have said since before my first book that we shouldn't have called it ADD/HD but rather CIS (Cultural Inconvenience Syndrome) because often the combination of brilliance and other issues made these kids culturally inconvenient and that is why medication is considered necessary.

What were the factors involved in the process of these individuals being created?

1. Expansion of access to the fuller capabilities of the brain.

2. A richer, better recorded, better shared history of what had gone before us, leading to the ability to expand the intellectual, emotional and physical understanding and interactions within the world.

3. The world becoming more connected therefore increased exposure to more and different ways of thinking and being in the world.

4. Decreased need for the majority of time and energy having to be devoted to simply surviving and daily living.

5. The cultural intermingling and expansion of an upper middle and a middle-middle class.

I have taken the following list of perspectives about ADD/HD from my first book. Bear in mind that I go into greater depth in the first book for each of these points. Also, at that time, no one was using ADD/HD, it was either A.D.D. and A.D.H.D and one of my suppositions was that the only difference was that A.D.H.D is simply A.D.D. on a bad diet and or in a bad environment or with other mitigating circumstances which were correctable, something which I still stand by. So anytime you see the term A.D.D. used in this book it is because it is an excerpt from the earlier book. However to use the language that will speak to the greatest number of individuals today, I simply use ADD/HD for this book.

1. ADD/HD is a *diff-ability,* not a disability.

2. ADD/HD is an indication of brilliance that the person must be taught how to access in order to utilize his/her full potential.

3. ADD/HD is a gift that is part of an evolutionary process.

4. The ADD/HD label has far-reaching and often negative effects upon the child labeled with it that is often not in the best interest of that child.

5. Easily changed or managed outside factors can have a profound effect on the ADD/HD person, meeting their goals without medication.

6. Due to the protocol used to diagnose individuals with ADD/HD, incorrect and/or incomplete diagnoses are a regular occurrence.

7. Diagnosis is often only pushed for in order to get the child medicated and the desire for a medicated child has more to do with convenience than the best interest of the child.

8. Medication is best used last, yet it is overused, recommended first and portrayed as the primary if not only option.

9. Medication hides or obscures other things which are potentially dangerous, harmful and, in some cases, life-threatening.

10. Isolation is one of the greatest risks for a person with ADD/HD. It is created from outside sources and, in and of itself, is not a tendency of ADD/HD, but of the environment. Unchecked isolation can lead a person who is brilliant to become emotionally unstable and potentially violent.

11. Depression is a dangerous side effect of ADD/HD. It can mask or mediate some of the more obvious signs of ADD/HD. Depression and medication achieve some of the same unhealthy results for the person with ADD/HD.

12. We risk our future through the 'drugging' of our children. If continued, this will lead to major upheavals, chaos and the destruction of our world, as we know it.

Verbiage Clarity

A great many words have multiple meaning. Phrases, colloquialisms and oxymoron's that change meanings throw further confusion into the mix. Add regional expressions, slang and tribal meanings, and it is amazing that we can communicate with each other at all. So often we think we know what someone else is saying only to find that they meant something different, sometimes a little different, sometimes a lot different. How many of you went back and read the sentence a second time that contained the phrase "tribal meanings" in it? In case you are wondering, I did not mean Native American meanings when I said "tribal meanings." What I mean is that we all have a "tribe" we belong to and one in which we grew up; sometimes one is an extension of the other, sometimes they blend and sometimes they are totally separate. We may even belong to more that one tribe or community. Your tribe growing up may have included your family, your school, your neighborhood (though not as often as it used to), church or any organizations to which you may have belonged. Within that tribe, or at least sections of that tribe, you may have had a very individualized slang that only people from the neighborhood or school really understood.

My point here is that there may be words or phrases that I use which have little or no meaning to you or a very different meaning. Because of the nature of my work and that I am working in a little understood area, when I started I created terms to express (sometimes as literally as possible) what was going on within the ADD/HD individual. I have tried to explain those as best I can along the way.

In the first book, I looked at the impact of ADD/HD from the perspective of four different levels; physical, emotional, intellectual and spiritual. I examined how we, as a species, had been operating at each of these levels, how the ADD/HD had impacted that level, why it was a gift and how to manage that gift. Here I have given the briefest of overviews to use as necessary reference points, as well as points of understanding to get the most out of this book.

Physical Energy Flow Patterns

Steady

The steady pattern is the energy pattern in which the individual will have an elevated energy level, but it is constant. The pattern will only become erratic when the person is forced (for long periods) to have no physical outlet for the energy.

Pulse

The pulse pattern is the energy pattern where the individual will have an elevated energy level, but many times the energy comes in pulses. The person will be more likely to fidget constantly whether he/she has been still for long periods or not.

Crescendo

The crescendo pattern is the energy pattern in which the individual's energy builds in a rhythm. The person will go from quiet, restful energy to increasingly frenetic until reaching a point where the person crashes and then returns to a resting energy state.

Emotional Patterns

The individual impacted by ADD/HD is more sensitive to the emotional energy around him. This person also tends to be more connected to those emotions. He is quite capable of emotional "flat lining" as well as having emotions in clusters or groups, which come in drops.

Because of the severity of the negative impact upon the child and the family that unmanaged or mismanaged emotional meltdowns have, I have included a section on a management tool to help with them.

Emotional Drops

Emotions do not flow in the traditional way in the ADD/HD child. When they experience events the emotional part gets withheld automatically, for processing later. Unlike children who withhold emotions due to fear or their inability to express emotions in a learned way, these children just hold onto them. They can collect several emotions at a time and if they don't make a concerted effort to process and release those emotions (or have to do so), they will have a "drop".

This happens in a variety of ways and rhythms. The withheld emotions create a ball of emotional energies that suddenly rush through the person's body.

Your child is then trying to deal with many, often times varied, emotions. If one were to think of emotions as one would think of colors of paints, when you mix too many what ends up happening is you get a very dark brown-black color and all the different colors become indistinguishable. In this case, think of the brown as frustration and the black as anger. Unless the drop happens with emotions (colors) that are all just variations on one or two primary colors, it becomes that dark brownish/black like something one would see pouring out of a sewer pipe. Depending on how many emotions there are and how charged they are, it can oftentimes be explosive when they are finally released. This to the observer is the "meltdowns" or temper tantrums often associated with these children. Meltdowns are simply the cleansing out of backed up emotions. The emotions can be their unreleased personal emotions or the emotions that they picked up along the way and have taken on. The meltdown happened because you or your spouse has been in a high anxiety or stressed state and your child keys into this and before you know it he is having the meltdown for you.

I have seen three primary variations of the drop pattern.

Hold-Drop

In the *Hold-Drop* pattern, the energies will be on hold until a certain number of emotions are reached and then they are dropped simultaneously into motion. I have seen the numbers range from 3 –18.

Squeeze, Hold-Drop

With the *Squeeze, Hold-Drop* pattern, some small part of the energy goes into motion, maybe 10-15%. In this pattern, the child has very understated emotions, whether positive or negative, to experiences around them. With the majority of the emotions being withheld for later processing. If the later processing doesn't happen, then those stored up emotions come out through a meltdown format

Hold-Drop with After-Shock

The last pattern I have detected has been one that has more to do with rhythm than anything else. In the first two patterns, there is a number which seems to trigger the release and when identified falls into a rhythm or pattern. With this one, the first number seems to be higher like a 13, 15 or even a 19 but after the drop there is a second drop after two, three or four.

Emotional Coffee Breaks

Now before I even explain this to you, I want you to understand that I have clients doing this. It can be done and it does help. I have clients from six to over sixty, who have had success with it. It takes some practice and you have to work with it. If you are more of an auditory or kinesthetic person then you may want to get my "Managing The Gift ™ Daily Practices CD," where on one of the tracks I actually walk you through doing a coffee break.

Emotional coffee breaks are just that, breaks, a time which is set aside on a regular basis for your child to process his emotions. The frequency of the breaks depends on his drop pattern.

In my first book, I discussed how this is an emotional body upgrade because of the amount of limitations and expectations we have put on the who, what, how, when and where of emotions. In today's world, emotional illness and emotionally created physical illness are the fastest growing categories of illness. We just don't do emotions well. After my first book on ADD/HD was out I was approached by an anger management therapist, who was working in the penal system, about how she used my emotional coffee break process on all her patients. After hearing her perspective that most people today do not process emotions in a healthy way, I began thinking of this process in wider terms. So before you can help your child have healthier emotions you want to check in on your own emotional health and self awareness level around your emotions. So I am going to begin by having you walk through the process, on a daily basis of doing an emotional coffee break for one month BEFORE you work with your child. So let's walk you through a coffee break.

In a nutshell, you go into the place where the energies are being held and bring them out one at a time. Have the emotion, decide what you need to do with the emotion, take any necessary action concerning the emotion and then let it go. You are basically draining off the emotions before they get a chance to drop on you.

This is how I have my clients create this:

1. Establish schedule based upon drop pattern.

2. When you have the coffee break, begin a mental review of everything which has transpired since your last review.

3. List any event that you know you would have had energy created on.

4. Review the event, what happened, what was said or done.

5. Intellectually decide what emotion or emotions would have been created.

6. Then go in and touch the emotion. Don't intellectualize it but touch it. Let your knowledge of how you know it feels lead you to the feeling.

7. If more than one feeling comes out around the issue make a list of all of them.

8. Acknowledge each and every one of them separately. Even allow yourself to say the feeling out loud, with the energy that is attached to it; i.e. *I feel hurt, or I feel angry.* Don't deadpan it; allow the feeling to flow out.

9. After you have honored and accepted all the individual feelings, associated with that event, then sort them by you & anyone else involved in the event, you & another person unrelated to the actual even, you & yourself, you and on old unresolved issue.

10. First decide on any action that you need to take with any person who was involved with the issue.

11. Next decide on any action that you need to take with another person, unrelated to the event but related to the feeling.

12. Then begin to process, maybe even journal on the other two aspects concerning feelings attached to the event.

13. Then, if you can't journal and work on the other two, schedule time that you can.

14. And if you feel that the issue is something that you can identify but don't know what or how to resolve it then find someone else to help you process it.

15. Move on to the next event. Repeat until done.

This may sound like a long, drawn out cumbersome process and will probably feel like it the first couple of times as well. But the more you do it the quicker, and clearer it becomes as to what is what and what you need to do about it. And the more that you do it the less other issues will be involved, because you will have cleared them out.

Emotional coffee breaks are just a version of a structured, goal-oriented time out. Instead of having to have a child do a time out because they had a meltdown, if you have them do a coffee break on a regular basis their meltdowns will become far less frequent.

Now you have completed your month of doing emotional coffee breaks on yourself, you now get to tailor the approach to your child depending on their age and ability to recognize their own emotions. I will go over the process for a young child and from there you can modify it for an older child. The goal is always getting your child to a point where they can do it for themselves. With a younger child you need to help them through the process and the process needs to be modified on the age and maturity level of your child but eventually they will learn how to have a preventive time out on their own, which is not a punishment instead of a time out for something they can't help, which more often than not is perceived as a punishment.

When working with younger children you simply begin the process by having them tell you about their day. Make a game out of it. After you have painted your child's portrait as described in the parenting chapter, how to get them to best communicate this information will be easier. Because of the tendency of the ADD/HD child to emotionally flat line you can't just sit back and look for emotional cues about how they were feeling, you actually have to be sharing your child's experience with them and then deduce whether the situations that they are speaking to you about are ones where some kind of emotion, that could get held in the emotional net, could have occurred. Then as they finish telling you about an incident ask them how they felt about that. If they seem to struggle with the concept of what they were feeling then offer them some insights to how they might have been feeling. This must be done very delicately as to not impose your feelings about the situation but help them figure out their feelings about the situation. When they have touched the feeling then let them feel it, perceive it and either breathe or do some kind of action to help them process through it. When that part is done then you move on to any possible teaching opportunity or an action/consequence example that can help your child grow and make shifts which may have avoided the situation in the past (if the emotion was negative) or draw more of those experiences to them (if the emotion was positive). Doing this after school, before bed or after a transition of some kind will help your child be more emotionally stable. Also your child should slowly begin to pick up the ability to do it on their own and then will only need to be prompted to do it. In my Daily practices CD, I walk children through a combination of shielding and an emotional coffee break in both the AM & PM meditation. Starting your child with those two and then delving deeper and helping with more emotional attachment and connection in the afternoon is a winning combination.

Intellectual Patterns

Individuals who have ADD/HD are accessing more of their brain, receiving and processing information differently. They tend towards a more kinesthetic learning style. They have a value-driven learning style. They also have a need for clear, unchanging truths. Their thoughts come in two primary patterns: *Spaghetti* or *Pulse/Burst*.

Spaghetti

Individuals with a spaghetti pattern have an endless array of thoughts constantly present and available within their consciousness. The minute they lose interest in whatever is in front of them, they have a multitude of choices regarding what they could be thinking. These people are often seen as the "dreamers."

Pulse/Burst

Individuals with a Pulse/Burst style receive thoughts in groups or clusters, often drawing their attention to a variety of different ideas and thoughts. If the cluster is so large that they actually stop for a moment or two and seem unable to respond or comprehend, then they are experiencing a burst of information.

This was not what I had run across when I wrote the first book in the "Managing the Gift" series. This does not surprise me, though, because I noticed shifts from generation to generation in people who were impacted with ADD/HD. Being a shift that is still in the process of evolving, I was also unsurprised to not find an adult with this pattern yet. I have named it DSL because at the time it was the fastest way to get information over the internet. Things change but I have kept the name the same. DSL is like the intellectual version of the steady pattern. The information just keeps flowing in, sometimes at a pretty quick rate. However, one does not necessarily have to pay attention to it. When in hyper focus mode, it is like a program that is just running in the background. With the spaghetti pattern, it is all just kind of there and new things will show up within the mind from which to choose, especially when what is going on outside the mind is of little or no interest. With the pulse and pulse/burst pattern, the information is popping in a way that can interfere with holding the attention on what is occurring outside the person's head, even when the person is interested. The DSL simply is nonstop, limitless information, of all varying levels and qualities. It has the best qualities of both but also has the drawback of getting so lost within the constant flow of information that the person with this style checks out to what is going on around him/her. It is almost like being in a self-induced coma of information.

The Spiritual Body: The ADD/HD Impact

The awareness of being more than just a physical body is one that, for the most part, comes naturally to the ADD/HD individual. They are more aware of their own energetic body and the energies that other people are putting out around them. They can be very sensitive and aware of other people's emotions, even when those emotions are not being expressed. They are able to pick up on negativity, disappointment, disapproval as well as true unconditional love, support and understanding. Oftentimes if they seem disconnected in their awareness, it is either due to their tendency to hyper-focus or as a type of self-protection mechanism. Anti-social behaviors help them from becoming overwhelmed by other people's emotions. They see themselves as here for some kind of purpose and know that they are here to make the world a better place. When they are allowed to touch it, both children and adults will speak of knowing that they are here for a greater purpose. Simply put, there are ways where they experience, see, perceive and interact with the world differently that the non- ADD/HD person does. Here are some of the things that a few of my clients have shared with me:

A twelve-year-old male child upon asking him what was "hurting" him in his life: "It hurts me to be human when I see what we have done, not only to each other, but to the planet itself. And I know I am here to make it better, but it hurts me to be human and see what we have done."

A thirteen-year-old male: "I know I have all this stuff, these gifts, that I am here to do something with. I just do not know how to get to them."

A nineteen year old male: "I cannot describe it, how I feel, but every time I see man do something destructive to the earth, it's like I feel the pain."

A forty-two year old woman: "I have always been so frustrated knowing I have all of these gifts to give the world and I just cannot seem to touch them enough to do it."

An eight-year old male: "I know I have to make the world a better place or soon there will not be an earth to be a better place."

A twenty-seven year old woman: "I am here to make a better world, I just wish people would stop trying to get in my way, and stop trying to limit me and medicate me because I do things differently. It's not my problem they do not understand."

A nine-year old boy: "I know I can have great power over people and I do not want to misuse it."

An eleven-year old boy when asked about why he had always hated guns as far back as anyone could remember: "I feel that way because of getting shot in the war and watching all my family getting killed before me—I hate war."

ADD/HD impacted people, as a group, seem to be more obviously and consciously aware of themselves as beings that have a spiritual nature. Many of the above comments have wisdom that one would expect from someone who had been consciously working on their path for some time, not someone who is eight or twelve or even nineteen years of age. Alongside this general awareness is a heightening of psychic/intuitive abilities. Like any individual who has been made uncomfortable with their own psychic abilities or has been "pushed" into denying them, ADD/HD impacted people might not be aware of these abilities. Once they are able to touch them and own them, however, look out! Empathy seems to be one psychic gift that is heightened somewhat in the majority of people with whom I have worked. Empathy is the ability to "feel" what someone else is feeling and sometimes even "take on" those feelings. This can leave the other person feeling better, while the ADD/HD impacted person has to now process through these feelings.

There are a number of other ways that the energetic body might play out the ADD/HD impact, but those would be more on a case by case basis. It boils down to an increase of awareness and an increase of abilities.

The Spiritual Body: Managing the Gift

Managing the gift of spiritually impacted ADD/HD people is by far the easiest of the four levels. It evolves around four basic concepts:

1. Help them learn how to shield and protect their personal energy.

2. Assist them in developing their own intuitive abilities.

3. Separate them from any limiting or judgmental concepts around spirituality.

4. Support them as spiritual beings.

The last is the easiest of the four. If you are supporting someone who is being impacted by ADD/HD, start by recognizing yourself as a spiritual being. See yourself as divinity on earth. For the impacted person, start an active exploration of a spiritual path. As you begin this process, remember that you redefine what spirituality can be. The same might hold true for many of the new things that will be introduced to you, not that this information will be right or wrong; it just will not be applicable to you. Because of the increase of spiritual awareness, helping the ADD/HD impacted person to see themself as a spiritual being is not a difficult task once you can break through their feelings of isolation. All of this depends, of course, on how spirituality has been portrayed to the person.

Help them learn how to shield and protect themselves

There are a number of different ways to protect and shield yourself so that you are not taking on other people's emotions or being sucked dry by other people. The book I would most recommend would be *Invisible Armor: Protecting Your Personal Energy* by Thomas Hensel. As long as there has been energy, there have been those that will dump the energy they do not want on whomever will take it and those that will suck any energy source they can access dry. You, as a person supporting an ADD/HD impacted person, need to learn about shielding and protection as well. This is to make sure that you are neither the one being sucked dry nor the one doing the sucking. Also, make sure that you are not taking on other people's stuff or putting your stuff onto other people.

More often than not, people are not aware of playing any of those roles. They feel the effect of playing the role, but they do not quite understand why they are feeling what they are feeling. Therefore, someone may feel drained after spending time with another person but not be able to quite put their finger on why. Alternatively, they may have emotions whirling around in them and not know where they came from. On the other hand, one can also know that they feel good, energized or powerful after exchanges with some people and not know why.

Depending on the level of impact on the emotional body, these feelings can be quite skewed. An empathic person does not necessarily have to create an emotion to feel a feeling. Emotion is energy in motion, and the energy is in motion as long as it has been catalyzed by an event. A feeling can be a sense of something. And a feeling can grow to the point where it can create an emotion, but it does not always *have* to create an emotion. The empathetic person can take on a feeling, a vague sensation, or they can take on an emotion, therefore needing to process the emotion that has been taken on. Sometimes the emotion will go into the emotional body hold/drop pattern and sometimes it will circumvent it. This will happen especially if the feeling is a vague feeling. These vague feelings can be the way in which their intuition may be speaking to them, throwing an additional consideration into the pot.

The isolation factor that often accompanies ADD/HD impacted people works in their favor. This is because the isolation can act as a type of shielding and protection; it is not a healthy kind, but it is a kind that will work. That is why it is important that, as the isolation becomes broken down, a healthier type of shielding is put in place. This will ensure that the person will not become overwhelmed.

Assist them in developing their own spiritual abilities

It is hard enough for average people who have not been brought up in an open and supportive environment to start the journey of being open to their spiritual selves. Oftentimes, ADD/HD impacted people have already felt different, like outsiders. Getting them to open up to their intuitive side can seem risky to them, like just another way they will not fit in.

Around the age of four or five, we start getting messages to discard any evidence of our spiritual being, at least the spiritual being which is showing itself in esoteric ways. Often, if a child is expressing past life memories, seeing energy fields, talking to dead people or if they "know" something they could not possibly know, then we start talking to them about "growing up" or "being a big boy or girl" and not making things up. We may also accuse them of lying. In some manner we communicate to them that what they are doing, sometimes even who they are, is wrong. We all know that children can be very imaginative, but we must be careful not to automatically dismiss everything that is not black and white by calling it "imagination." It is also making sure that you are not trying to dismiss or eliminate the behavior because it makes you, the adult, uncomfortable or requires you to shift your perspective or stretch your comfort zones. It is often said that children are our greatest teachers, so let them be. For ADD/HD impacted adults, encourage them to go out onto the limb. Encourage them to read, take classes and find someone with whom to work who will help them discover and own themselves as spiritual beings.

In this review, I have basically tried to bring you "up to speed" by using some highlights from the first book in this series. More points from the first book will be utilized, as appropriate, throughout the book.

Closing Thoughts Before We Move Forward... Pros and Cons: ADD/HD

I have been accused of romanticizing ADD/HD. That I want to put these individuals up on a pedestal and that I do not see them for all the trials and tribulations that they can cause, for themselves and others. Some people only like to focus on the inconvenient side of the impact that the ADD/HD child can be:

- Inattentive

- Distractible

- Restless

- Impulsive

- Disorganized

- Hyperactive

- Argumentative

- Compulsive

- Pessimistic

- Quick Temper

- Period of panic and fear

- Forgetful

- Difficulty with follow through

- Poor internal supervision

And here are some of the gifts of ADD/HD that when better understood and managed actually not only eliminate many of the problems but help bring humanity to its next level of existence:

- Brilliant
- Creative/Artistic
- Outside the box thinking
- Rebellious
- Justice/fairness orientated
- High energy
- Loves to learn
- Loves to teach
- Inventive
- Compassionate

All a matter of perspective, isn't it?

CHAPTER 2

PARENTING

The Evolving Parent

PARENTING IS AN evolving job. Children don't come in with an owner's manual. You can only look back and primarily all you know about parenting is how you were parented: good, bad and indifferent. You can read, study and remember those friends who had parent's you wished you had, or didn't, as perhaps other indicators of what to do or not do but the default will always be the parent's and parented experiences you had from your own childhood. What parents discover all too soon, is children are not smaller versions of their parents and they aren't who the parent was as a child. Also, the parents' job is not to be who their parents were as parents, no matter how good at parenting we felt they were. The parenting is happening 20 to 40 years later, at a different time and place, in a different culture with different children that have different needs. Just as the world has evolved, so have the demands of parenting evolved. So as you read this book, remember, no one is served by using the information that it contains as a way to beat yourself about what a bad parent you are. It is all too easy to go to the default of what we know, which is why we suddenly find ourselves saying the same phrases that our parents said that we hated. But just because we can now understand why they might have said it, doesn't mean that it is automatically the best thing to say (or do). Our parents job as parents was to bring us as far along as they were capable of doing. Our job as parents is to pick up where they left off and to bring it to a higher level of parenting, not to replicate.

Rather, than beat yourself up, let me give you the best skills possible and then when you don't apply it, don't make it a big deal. It's not going to be the end of their life. Let's continually say I want you to apply more and more of the right language, the correct skills, and do the things that are going to most help your child. This is what it means to be an evolving parent.

The role of the parent is to help a child come into and then navigate life, assisting the child to become his highest self. A parent's responsibility includes helping the child to discover, understand, embrace and lovingly accept himself. It is the parent's role to provide not only physical safety but also to promote emotional health, mental development and an attitude that includes a sense of being part of the larger whole. This includes learning to function within their day-to-day social structure, understanding their role in the local community, and gaining a sense of their place in the greater world. This includes some perception of a larger self, God, or divine being. Also, the parent should function as both the child's advocate to the world and protector from it. Then, there is the more mundane side of parenting as well, such as running the household, pursuing a career and maybe even trying to have some kind of personal life. Yes, I did say personal life, because parents who do not take care of themselves end up running out of the energy to do what must be done for everyone else.

So what does a parent of the child who they believe may have ADD/HD do?

First and foremost, even if you are certain your child has ADD/HD, do not rush to get an official diagnosis. Weigh the pros and cons. Look at the child's age. Examine what assistance has been put in place for the child and what are the actual issues that require the diagnosis? How is it going to serve your child to have that diagnosis? Remember that labels are often easier to get than to get rid of.

Second, has your child asked for help? Is your child struggling or is it the people around him who are asking for help? Keep in mind that if you are trying to help a child who does not perceive that there is a problem, you will end up giving him one. When this occurs, it most often makes the child's ability to receive assistance more difficult in the long run. The sooner your child feels like something is wrong with him, the sooner there *will* be, even if there was no problem to begin with.

So your child, whether labeled or not, seems to be struggling with focus, with controlling their energies and maybe even with unexpected, sudden or out of control meltdowns, where do you start?

Shifting Behaviors

Unfortunately children do not come with an instruction manual. This means that more often than not, parents are left to rely on the methods and phrases used by their own parents. Unfortunately, those methods were not always healthy or constructive. Here are two such approaches to parenting which can do more harm than good.

Emotionally Based Approach

Emotional appeals or emotionally punishing your child's behaviors create long-term emotional issues for him regarding self-love and can interfere with his ability to be in healthy relationships in adulthood. Some examples of this kind of parenting are statements such as:

1. "If you really loved me, you wouldn't act that way."

2. "When you behave like that it makes it hard on your father and I."

3. "How do you think it makes me feel when the teacher calls and tells me you've been misbehaving in class?"

4. "It's harder to love you when you act up."

These statements express to your child emotional withdrawal and angry attacks which link your love of him to being dependent on his behavior. This puts the responsibility of your emotions onto your child when they are your own. It also begins the journey of conditional love. The child then begins to wonder "under what conditions will my parents love me, more, less or not at all?"

What makes this emotional pattern set-up even more insidious is when the conditions which make the child feel unlovable are things that they have no control over. An example of this I see all the time is a parent rewards or bribes the child with a food based treat which is guaranteed to create a sugar high and then a sugar crash. When the sugar high hits its peak the child is hyper and out of control. The parent then punishes the child for the behavior, which the child can't help in the moment, because they are on a sugar high. Then the sugar crash happens and the child acts out in a different way, receives another kind of punishment or berating which is filled with conditional love statements, again something the child could not help in the moment, as they were coming down. The child does not understand about the behavior. The behavior was instigated through a parental choice and the child had no control over the behavior in the moment and yet was punished for it.

Oftentimes in trying to guide and support your child you may use emotional manipulation making them responsible for how you feel or experience their behavior. However, the expression of emotion needs to be based on your *child's experience* of the situation rather than your own. An example of this is:

1. "It makes me sad when you don't have a good day at school because I know it upsets you."

2. "It makes me happy when you have a good day. How can we help you to have a better day?"

These statements do not reflect any particular inadequacy on your child's part or that your child's behavior negatively effects your feelings which could result in your child feeling shame.

Assigning Value Approach

Avoid tying your child's value or intrinsic self worth to concepts of good and bad based on their actions. Using the phrases "good boy/bad boy" as a way to encourage good behavior and discourage bad behavior links their actions to their value as a person which often leads to self-worth issues and an inability to love themselves and allow others to love them later in life. These labels of "good and bad" oftentimes seem to not apply or make sense to your child and therefore are not easily integrated. It is better to focus on the effort they put into the situation (i.e. grades) rather than the actual outcome.

The problem with good/bad and emotionally based parenting is that you are making children responsible for something that they cannot truly comprehend. What they do get out of the mix, however, is that they are bad people and that your love is conditional. The "I am angry at your actions not at you" motif can only be effective if the experience can be tied to an action/consequence model that leads to making better choices and developing critical thinking skills.

Over-Praising

Praise, praise, praise; never criticize! Some people will tell you that this way of thinking is the way to go; I say it is a load of hooey. Of course we want to recognize when the child has done something particularly well, just as we want to constructively critique, in a loving and positive way, when they have not. We are now seeing a generation of young adults who have a hard time making it in the real world because they fall apart at the first sign of criticism, no matter how well done. This is also a generation that struggles to function unless they are told constantly how good they are or how great whatever they did was. We have handicapped these young adults through the mistake of over-praising, which then loses meaning that combined with a lack of constructive criticism, which is what helps them to improve, sets them up for failure. They emerge into the adult world wearing rose-colored glasses, and those glasses are being shattered left and right causing chaos in the workplace and oftentimes leaving them unable to cope in the real world.

Actions and Consequences

I would like to think that actions and consequences would speak for themselves, but unfortunately in my years of working with families, ADD/HD and not, the concept of actions and consequence just becomes a convoluted way to say punishment. In order for action-consequence parenting to really be effective, actions have to be consistently linked in the mind of the child to their resulting consequences. There must be even-handed energy applied to the consequences of all actions that have obvious consequences (such as carrying a milk cup to the table so it doesn't spill), until the child has truly integrated the concept.

To utilize action-consequence parenting effectively, everyone's involvement in modeling the concept is also important. When an older sibling or even a parent receives clearly desirable or undesirable consequences as a result of their actions, those opportunities should be used as teaching tools. As the child develops better critical thinking skills and more maturity, the subtleness of actions and consequences needs to be stressed. For instance, making the connection between staying up too late the night before and being tired the next day and therefore having a bad day.

Also, avoid absolutes (not everyone who breaks the law gets caught or punished) and concede that there are people who do get away with inappropriate behavior. Provide examples of how actions and their consequences affect the family, community, and the immediate and greater world as your child's maturity and experiences allow comprehension. With these children, do not be afraid to challenge them to rise to the next level of thinking and understanding.

I recently was going to church with a client of mine, a mother of three, one of which is an ADHD child. On the way there, she interactively went through what the expectations were to be in church with her young ADHD child, questioning and engaging him as to how much he remembered on his own and what she really needed to remind him concerning the proper behaviors in church. She covered things such as noise, the appropriate volume of singing, as well as staying quiet while the minister was praying and prompted her child as to why. She also explained the consequences of not adhering to that behavior and reminded him how certain behaviors made certain things happen and how other behaviors led to other consequences, in a language he could understand. The child was five. Was his behavior perfect? No, but it was impressively acceptable. The child was allowed to fidget in the pew, draw on a piece of paper and was rewarded with a thank-you every time he showed he participated in the appropriate behaviors. Would have the mother rather been chatting with me, or just singing, or praying or listening to the sermon? Sure, but she did what it took to be the kind of mother her child needed and because she prompted him in advance, went over actions and consequences and then prompted him with thank-yous and reminders when necessary, she got to do a whole lot more of the things she wanted to be doing rather than engaging in a battle of the wills.

Battles of the Wills

Do not bother. For every battle you win, there will be additional ones created that you will lose. The reason your ADD/HD child can become stubborn leading to a battle in the first place is because he has so many thoughts and ideas in his head like a rushing river going 90 miles an hour. So, when he makes a decision about something as being true he creates a mooring post of that piece of information which is within the rushing river as a truth he can count on. This now becomes something which allows him to be able to take a mental break from the continuous onslaught of intellectual possibilities which exist in relation to that information. This delicate matrix of "truths" is used to create some kind of stability in his life. Therefore, simply telling your child that he is wrong about something upsets his mental apple cart. This opens him back up to the possibility of having to question everything.

When your child does become stubborn about something, you need to work through his logic process with him and figure out where his is stuck or where there has been a misunderstanding between the two of you. Ask a series of open ended questions such as "Why is that?" and "Talk to me about how you came to that conclusion." Try to create an atmosphere where your child can be completely honest no matter how crazy his answer may seem to you.

Obviously this process will not help a lot with children whose age is at either side of the logic spectrum. If they are too young, they do not have the skills for the conversation, and when they hit teenage years, their logic can be illogical. However, if you have created a communication style of inclusion and mutual participation that implements encouragement and critical thinking skills, your teenager will be more logical than his average peer.

Increasing Focus Through Diet

Children don't understand the ramifications of what they eat and how it plays out in how they feel and act. They must be taught. Luckily ADD/HD children are bright, and through a combination of dialogue and critical-thinking based interactions about foods using the action and consequence method of parenting, they can and will become self-monitoring.

Also remember that children learn more by what they observe than by what they are told. If you are a person who desires the freedom to eat whatever you want without accepting the ramifications for what you are eating, then working with your kids regarding diet is going to be difficult.

If your child is being regularly exposed to people who have extremely obvious food-related issues, such as weight problems and/or very poor diets, those issues must be discussed in a manner which is age appropriate for the child. Without being judgmental, you can use the action and consequence methodology when explaining the negative impact of eating foods that are either just plain unhealthy or simply do not agree with you.

There are some foods for the ADD/HD child which are incompatible with their physical system. This can result in some low level of what I would call an "allergic reaction" to these foods. These physical irritants lead to them to an experience in which they become uncomfortable in their own skin leading to undesirable behaviors such as an inability to focus, hyperactivity or meltdowns. Unfortunately, it seems that only in extreme cases, when faced with actual pain, ticks, or skin disruptions, do people think allergic reaction. However, when the allergic reaction is more subtle, people can easily dismiss it. Things like meltdowns, tantrums, hyperactivity, and an inability to focus do not necessarily trigger in us the thought that this could be a form of allergic reaction to foods or even environment.

Several years ago, shortly after I began working with ADD/HD adults and children on a regular basis, a young man with whom I was working with turned out to have an issue with wheat. It was one of the contributing factors to his "over the top" ADD/HD behavior. He was also diagnosed with Tourette's syndrome. At the age of nine, he was not thrilled with it but he was willing to go on a wheat-free diet. Within weeks, his ability to focus increased, his excessive energy level became more manageable and he stopped having the tics that one often associates with Tourette's. Though he was not happy with this change in his diet, he much preferred to not have tics, which were making him self-conscious. He was less aware of the improvements regarding his focus and energy, as were the people around him, but all were happy that he was getting in less trouble. Then he went away for Memorial Day weekend to his grandparents, who insisted that it was cruel to him to be unable to eat like the other kids, so by the time he arrived home the issues were all slowly beginning to return. However, everyone just reasoned it away ("Summer is coming," etc.).

Before we knew it, the child was back where he started. His lack of what was perceived as a tangible, serious reaction seemed to nullify the obvious results. Besides, as his grandparents mentioned, what's wrong with him just taking his medication?

Now, before you run out and take wheat out of your child's diet, wheat might not be the problem. It could be dairy, food dyes, highly refined chemically-processed foods or even high fructose corn syrup. The list of things that I see which occur regularly as contributors to exacerbating and difficult-to-deal-with ADD/HD behavior, goes on and on. Yes, there are some common things worth checking into. I have just named a few.

My point is to not underestimate the power of both eliminating things out of your child's diet and adding things into it. Just as with removing harmful things from one's diet, I have found that adding in certain nutrients can also make a tremendous difference.

Remember, however, to view working with diet as something that is part of a larger protocol to help you better access all the gifts that come with ADD/HD and manage the challenges; it is not the final solution. Diet is not the only thing that needs to be addressed. Oftentimes people approach the diet issue from just a simple "don't eat" approach without understanding what the issue really entails. Thus, the positive effects that could be realized are not.

Later in the book, there will be additional discussion of this issue.

Play

Play is important; play structure is more important. Keep a young child away from computers and televisions as much as possible. There are aspects of both watching TV and being on the computer that simulate motion and give the sensation of the release of physical energy without the actual releasing of the energy. This affects his ability to go to sleep and his ability to remain calm when being calm is required for certain activities. Structuring play to make it as physical, kinesthetic and critically-thinking based as possible allows the play to engage the mind and release the energies while the child develops the ability to be more self-policing.

Play is also an important part of developing the child's mind. It directly correlates with his ability to be social and develop healthy tenacity and physical awareness, and along the way play helps him find joy in learning and promotes his own natural curiosity. Also, play that does not center itself around computers and TV can also help to develop better critical-thinking skills and imagination, and help with motivation.

Body and Energy Awareness

One of the best ways to help your child is to first come to an understanding within yourself. Given the complex nature of the interplay between energy, emotions and the body, it is important for you, the parent, to have your own awareness. This will help you to be able to help your child with their own emotions. Emotions are just energy-in-motion or e-motions.

Next time you have a very intense emotion, good or bad, stop and ask yourself where exactly you feel it. It may radiate within your whole body but it may only be located within a specific spot. Sometimes this location shifts but often they reside in the same places. When you can identify them and connect with them in your mind then you can ask yourself why you are having that feeling and what is it about. Then you get to make choices about that feeling and whether you choose to manage the feeling and figure out how to be productive with it or let the feeling manage your life and therefore create an undesirable reality or consequence.

By the time a child is three or four, he can start to become consciously aware of the energies and emotions within his body. The child can actually find where excess energies and emotions are building. These energies must be connected, within the child's awareness, as leading to behaviors and consequences that are undesirable. Without a sense of ownership or "buy-in", and being given the opportunity to make the connection within their own reality, these children can become overwhelmed which pushes them to become rigid, stubborn and inflexible. They know what they are "supposed to do", but they cannot seem to remember or to bring it together because the connection has not been made within them.

Unwilling Willing Disobedience

If you will forgive the pun, in "unwilling willing disobedience" it is as if the brain has a mind of its own and with these individuals that may just be the reality of it. As pliable, agreeable and wanting to please as some of these children (and adults) that I have worked with have been, they still can not seem to retain certain pieces of information, perhaps chores they need to do, activities they agreed to participate in or something they promised to learn and simply could not. Without exception, the child (or adult) forgot or broke promises because the value proposition was more someone else's than their own. As much as they wanted to please or make the other person happy, to the "mind" part of the brain, what was being asked was of little or no interest or value and until this was established the individual failed far more often than they succeed at whatever the promise or agreement was. Somehow the "do it because I told you to", the "do it because I will punish and/or reward you for it" and especially the "do it because you love me" just does not cut it for that mind. The mind that runs the brain from a subconscious level determines what is important, interesting and has value. Sometimes the value proposition can only be achieved through experience(s).

One mother with whom I worked with was very frustrated because she had to constantly hound and follow-up on her child to brush his teeth when he was at an age where she felt he should be self-responsible enough to do it on his own. She would get frustrated and either end up yelling at him or removing this or that privilege. The problem was that, upon talking to the child, bad breath (which caused people to make fun of him), cavities, and toothaches had not yet come into his reality. Brushing teeth was something he was indifferent to unless his mouth tasted bad and that could be solved just as easily by eating or drinking something. He hated his mother yelling at him and it upset him to upset her, but on some level it was her problem, not his. Let me state clearly here that this feeling was not on a conscious level. Because of his processing and learning styles we started by giving him a project where he had to research and present to us the relationship between brushing and oral problems. Because we presented the project in a way that caught his interest, he did it. His brushing habits became somewhat better but still were not where they needed to be. However, he finally did end up with a cavity and toothache, and had to go through the process of having it fixed. After linking this unpleasant experience with his brushing habits and the information he had found out on his own, his mother never had to talk to him about brushing his teeth again. He wanted to do the right thing, but until he could have his "mind" convinced of its value, the brain simply did not retain the idea of brushing his teeth.

I have watched "unwilling willing disobedience" play out in hundreds of ways with my ADD/HD clients. When I have shared this concept with other people who have worked with this population and they think about it, they begin to see it clearly as well. Depending on other factors going on in the child's life, such as stress level and the amount and kind of support he is getting, this behavior could shift into what appears as oppositional defiant behavior.

Another thing to consider is what might best be called a safety issue. It is not uncommon for the default answer to be no when asked to do or to think about anything. That is more likely to happen if your child has an external processing style. We will go into processing styles and how to best work within them later. For the internal processing style they are more likely to say yes and then simply not do it. This happens because "no" or not taking the desired action creates no change. Yes means that are potentially opening up to a new set of experiences where they may not know what the expected behaviors or responses will be or whether or not in that moment they will be capable of them.

Advocate

As a parent, you get to be an advocate to the outside world for your child through making their educational, health and social decisions, which includes knowing when to fight for them and when to fight with them. It is important to understand a few key points about the effects and impacts of ADD/HD to determine if what is being asked of them and the way that it is being asked is understandable to and doable by them. Also, it is imperative to weigh the pros and cons of the situation as well as determine whether what is being asked is in the best interest of the child or in best interest of the party/parties that are asking.

Keep a journal of your observations about your child. Look for the answers to the following questions:

1. Are there rhythms to any meltdowns your child may have?

2. Are there things you know will trigger your child?

3. What are the things you have used that have been most successful in helping your child when he gets stuck?

4. What motivates your child?

5. Where and when is your child most likely to get overwhelmed and lost?

Later on in the book, you will expand the above list of questions plus work with additional information to "paint your child's portrait" which will assist you as you help your child, and improve your child's support systems.

CHAPTER 3

SIDE EFFECTS OF BEING ADD/HD IN A NON-ADD WORLD

ANOTHER THING TO be aware of for your child is the impact on him of being different in a world where differences are not always treated well. The structures that children participate in were created to serve the average child. Your child is not the average child, and in many cases those institutions no longer even serve the average child very well. Some side effects to watch for are low self-esteem, low self-worth, depression, anxiety and stubbornness, resistance to change, shame, fear and isolation.

Low Self-Esteem

I view self-esteem and self-worth as two different things. Though they are often used interchangeably, understanding the difference between the two can help determine where the problem may lie and how it can best be fixed. When a person is held in great esteem, he is recognized for the things he has accomplished. When one has low self-esteem one questions one's ability to achieve. That may or may not affect how a person perceives his value. If your child has low self-esteem, he may have an unwillingness to try things or is always assuming that he will fail. This low self-esteem may play out in a single area, such as music. Your child has been told or is convinced that he can never play a musical instrument or even be musical; he has low self-esteem in that area. In another area (computer games for example), your child may thrive and be very confident. He may have a high self-esteem in relation to computer games. This may or may not be transferable to other things he perceives that he does well or feels others perceive that he does well.

If your child has low self-esteem in an area:

1. Try to understand why he has decided to value that area, remembering that he will not have low self-esteem issues surrounding something that he does not value or ascribe importance to. Your child will not succeed at something that he does not perceive as having personal value and therefore does not berate himself for not achieving success in that area.

2. After understanding why that particular thing is valuable to him, connect the dots between that and something at which he is naturally gifted where there may be some cross over from which he can draw to become better at the subject at hand.

3. Choose a common task or interest that your child would like to be successful with. Create a game plan to which he commits based on the idea that it is important to him. Break that plan into manageable pieces that allow for frequent opportunities for success.

4. Constantly reinforce those small milestones to ensure that your child builds enough confidence so that when he does reach his intolerable frustration level, he is more apt to push through the wall and continue through to success.

5. Check in along the way to make sure that he hasn't lost interest and is only trying to succeed to please you. On the other hand make sure that he isn't just giving up because he thinks that he is incapable.

ADD/HD people are notorious for not finishing things. This occurs because once they have reached a level of mastery in whatever they are doing and are content with that level, they do not see the value of wasting their time to just be able to say that they finished. Also, unfinished projects can be used as positive distractions that can be used to help when the ADD/HD mind needs to be engaged on a surface level so it can work something out on a deeper level.

However, once the ADD/HD mind knows it can finish something or has gotten the bulk of the challenge or fun out of something, it does not have the same attachment to finishing things as the greater world does.

Low Self-Worth

A person's overall value is affected when low self-worth occurs. It includes self-concepts such as "I am a failure/loser" and "I can't do anything right." The "I can't do anything right" mentality belongs to a person who is struggling with both low self-esteem and low self-worth. A child can have great self-esteem surrounding something that he has found value in. But if your child perceives that the "powers that be" find no value in it and that everything that is considered valuable he "stinks at", then this feeling moves him towards low self-worth. This is the place where children get confused regarding the difference between their actions and themselves as individuals. Our emphasis on traditionally measured success, which oftentimes is not a measure of intelligence for the ADD/HD mind, sets these kids up to feel stupid. These children then use their stupidity, inability to focus and/or to remember, as manipulation tools. This often begins early in life when the things that are most emphasized as having value are things which seem beyond their grasp to understand or complete. As they go into increasingly more structure situations, day care and then preschool, a low sense of worth can be reinforced, depending on how their differences are handled. Certainly by the time they are exposed to a pass/fail system, followed by a grading system they can easily be struggling with self-worth issues. These struggles happen both in social-emotional situations, as well as academic-intellectual situations. Depending on how situations such as losing interest in finishing a project or a playdate meltdown are handled can impact the child's view of their own value or worth.

When you see signs of your child showing self-worth issues you also want to examine what their school experiences have been to date. If it is clear that their grades are not an accurate representation of their intelligence or their understanding of the material, then you may need to advocate for the implementation of different ways in which competence and the understanding and utilization of what they are learning is measured. Do not let people use outdated or incorrect measurement tools to assign your child's value in their mind or your mind and especially not in your child's mind.

Depression

One day, I began to notice a pattern of depression among the people with whom I was working. At first, I felt that it was probably just related to the isolation, fear, anxiety and shame factors that I addressed. However, I began to notice that the adults who had created techniques to deal with the impacts of the ADD/HD or those who were on medication still tended to lean towards pessimism and could easily fall into obvious depression. The more I looked, the more I saw thought processes and actions that could create or draw depression to them. When they began to see that they were always in trouble, nothing but trouble and tested or showed poorly in traditional academic ways, they would give up even trying.

I began to look at the love affair with depression. How did it serve them? What made it useful? I often ask these questions in the empowerment work that I do. What I realized was that depression can be a form of self-medication.

Depression literally depresses or shuts the person down, affecting energy level and motivation. Someone who is overactive and thinks too much and thus stands out as a result could easily look *normal* if all those symptoms were *depressed.* I am not saying that the ADD/HD impacted person makes a conscious decision to become and stay depressed; however, because of many of the things that are occurring in his life, ADD/HD people are very susceptible to getting depressed. The cycle can begin there.

The cycle could easily look like the following example in which we will name our case example Katie. After struggling with feeling outside, different, broken, disabled, and in general a problem to the people in her life, Katie finally succumbs to depression. She becomes more subdued. She talks less and is less hyperactive. She may even seem less distracted. She may not be a great deal more attentive, but she is less obviously distracted and she is certainly less disruptive. Now, someone with keen insight may approach Katie and ask her if she is okay because she is not acting like herself. On the other hand, she may also be rewarded for what appears to be better behavior. Katie may have had a hard time falling asleep or had an irregular sleeping pattern and because of this, getting up in the morning was a real chore. Now she is sleeping more than she ever did and, though she is not thrilled with mornings, she seems to put up fewer struggles about getting up. She appears to have resigned herself to this new pattern. In reality, Katie is just feeling too defeated to fight about it.

Ultimately Katie is perceived as doing better and is praised. She starts to feel better and the depression lightens up. Guess what happens? Katie starts perking up. She starts acting more like old Katie. Someone who is really tuned in is likely to welcome back the old, true Katie. However, an equally possible if not more likely scenario, is one where Katie hears that it was "too good to last." She may be asked, "What happened? You were doing so well." Katie prefers the way she was being treated when she was depressed and she may even try to recreate the behavior. Without something suppressing the extra energy, without something suppressing the wonderfully curious and constantly going "mind", she is unable to achieve that behavior. Katie starts feeling hopeless and negative, the depression returns and the cycle has started. After a few times through the cycle, the balance created is that of someone who tends towards pessimism and is mildly depressed or, at the very least, given to depression. That depression then becomes a nice, safe, cozy place to hang out. Depending on how big the swings are, this person could easily appear manic-depressive. I am not going to say that this happens to every ADD/HD impacted person. However, it is a scenario that can happen and may happen more often than anyone realizes.

One young man with whom I was working often talked about his lifetime struggle with pessimism and depression. He would talk about how he could sleep eighteen hours a day. He wanted a cat's life. However, when he would get involved with certain creative projects, those that would require many of his ADD/HD gifts, he would become brilliant, outgoing and friendly, functioning on very little sleep for weeks while working on the project. His pessimism would disappear and there were no signs of depression. He was allowed to have (and was even embraced for) his *artistic temperament.*

When I began working with him, he was in-between projects, dealing the best he could in a world that did not allow for his highly energized, artistic temperament. I shared with him my theories regarding ADD/HD, especially focusing on the one about depression. I told him that, as we worked with some of the protocols and gave him some new perspectives, he might find that his pessimism and depressive nature would shift. He might even need less sleep. The thought of sleeping less did not really appeal to him, but the rest of it did, so we gave it a shot. Within six months, he was sleeping less, was more optimistic and was not feeling depressed. He also had not worked on any of the artistic projects that had been a haven for him in the past. He discovered that he could function in both worlds and could allow himself to be artistic everywhere. He could even be a little temperamental, but not detrimentally so.

From a diagnostic perspective oftentimes the link between ADD/HD and depression is completely overlooked. The ADD/HD person who is mildly depressed ends up hearing the great pronouncement that they are outgrowing their ADD/HD. That could be because the mild depression acts like medication, or perhaps because the person has developed ways to not stand out negatively. The person may have also developed tools to make things work. Inside, the person knows they have not changed. Maybe the person has tried to convince themself that they have outgrown it, but they know that it is simply not true. Whatever the case, if your child's ADD/HD has seemed to have gone away but they are withdrawn, less excited about things, and have lost their rebellious nature and you have not been medicating them, then you may want to check in with them and see if they have given up and are struggling with depression. Make sure they are not being rewarded for feeling bad about who they are and/or being depressed.

When you cannot determine why you are depressed, at least not in a way you can express, it is far too easy to decide that it must be chemical or that it must be hereditary and would be best dealt with through medication. Having parts of yourself that you cannot seem to get your hands around makes all kinds of addictions easy — depression being one of those addictions. Therefore, if you or a loved one suffers with depression and has ADD/HD, think carefully about applying the techniques and perspectives is this book. When you find you have nothing to hide and nothing about which to be ashamed, you may find depression is a great deal less attractive a companion.

Stubbornness and Resistance to Change

It can appear as though ADD/HD children struggle with change and can be very stubborn. One of the main reasons for this is that they experience the world in such a different way than the people around them. Often they have set themselves up for negative feedback or consequences when they do something new or they do something differently than they have done before. This creates anxiety about being able to manage the change.

When they know that something is going to happen, they can prepare for it. They can think it through and get comfortable, making it less likely that their response will be viewed as unacceptable.

Another reason that change is difficult for them to navigate is that they can be overwhelmed by external energies coming from other people and the environment around them. Not being mentally prepared for them can lead to either a physical or emotional meltdown.

Ways to Deal With Anxieties Over Change

1. Help them visualize what will happen as a result of this change. Help them picture how things are going to be different than before.

2. Have them talk through the anxieties and see them as colors or shapes within their bodies and then get rid of them within their minds.

3. Focus them on some "general" specifics about the upcoming situation that draw on familiar situations from their past.

4. Teach them to ground and protect themselves.
   (If these are techniques that you are unfamiliar with I teach them in both my CD's and DVD's.)

A third reason why they tend to cling to the known involves the amount of things that are going on in their heads. There is a constant flood of thoughts, ideas, and feelings that are always pouring into ADD/HD children. They have to think about what is known much less than they do something that still needs processing. Once they have actually come to a conclusion about something, they cling to it, for to change it is to take it from a nice strong "know," like a mooring of truth in a rapid river of change, and push it back out into the river. This also plays out in what appears to be an inability to be wrong. Even when they can clearly see that they are wrong they will still hold onto an idea or a concept rather than throw it back out into that rapid river of thoughts and feelings.

Many of them reach a point where they have been perceived as being wrong so often that they cannot emotionally handle being wrong again. Their history of being wrong usually begins when they are young and they do not always have the vocabulary or the sentence structure to clearly communicate what is going on in their head. Their passion and excitement in trying to communicate their inner landscape can often come across as if they are skipping steps. Sometimes they can end up talking in half sentences or having the information come out in a jumbled way. The damage to their psyche is increased if they are overly exposed to a black and white, simple yes or no environment, (which is made doubly worse if they are an external processor) instead of an environment where they are guided and supported to put their jumbled thoughts in order. Sooner or later they can often simply just shut down and stop trying at all.

Here is the best way to deal with the "I can't be wrong" syndrome:

1. When you do need to correct your child, do not approach him with any reference to his being wrong.

2. Ask your child to clarify his answer because you do not understand how he came to that conclusion.

3. Explore your child's logic sequence that led to his erroneous conclusion. How did he get to the answer he gave or question that he asked?

4. When you find the piece of information that was not heard or comprehended correctly, assure your child that you can certainly understand how he reached that conclusion with that particular interpretation of the information.

5. If the logic based on the facts that your child heard is good and solid, make sure you praise him for getting an answer that made sense based on the assumptions with which he was working.

6. Correct the piece of information without casting blame on how the piece of information was misconstrued.

7. Come up with the corrected answer with him (if he does not do it on his own once the information was corrected) and celebrate arriving at the right answer.

8. If the piece of information was incorrect, misunderstood, or misheard because of your child's lack of attention during the process, then apply a combination of critical thinking skills within the actions and consequences model._During the whole process, do not attack him for not listening or for messing up again. Try not to show signs of frustration. None of those actions will help correct the behavior and will only move him towards giving up more easily next time or choosing not to even bother.

Anxiety

There are a number of different reasons why anxiety can run high within this group. We already went over some of the anxiety that can be caused as a result of change. Another circumstance in which a child can become anxious is when he is in a highly emotional situation. This can cause anxiety because the child is picking up on stress and anxiety around them. When the child goes into a hyper-focus mode he tends to be oblivious to what is going on around him. However, when the child comes into a new situation or for some reason needs to be fully present in a current situation, he can pick up on the emotional disturbances around him, which creates anxiety within himself leading to meltdowns and bad behaviors.

The ADD/HD child displays other anxieties surrounding their fears of unknowingly doing something which garners negative responses from the people around them. Those responses may arise from feeling anger and frustration at being made fun of or being viewed as a failure. Because memorizing things or even remembering things which have not been connected with either value or meaning to the ADD/HD "mind", it is a consistent issue that the child does not act, perform or behave well in prescribed socially acceptable manners. That can lead to him being ostracized from peers and excluded from activities because adults do not want to deal with the child's behavior.

Isolation

The inward focus of ADD/HD children is a common occurrence which stems from the fact that they are overwhelmed by all that is going on in their "minds". They are trying to make sense of both the internal as well as external stimuli. Often these children are more sensitive to their physical and energetic environment and are not in touch with their own meltdown points. Also, because they are likely to miss social cues, they do not fit in well with their peers during unsupervised social play. Therefore, there can be a tendency to isolate unless they can find one or two close friends with whom they deeply connect.

Shame and Guilt

According to cultural anthropologist Ruth Benedict, shame is a violation of cultural or social values. [2] Because of the nature of these children, they often do not comprehend social nuances or see the importance of social values especially ones that do not make sense or seem to have no purpose. This does not, however, stop the child from being affected by social out-casting. Psychoanalyst Helen B. Lewis argues, "The experience of shame is directly about the self, which is the focus of evaluation. In guilt, the self is not the central object of negative evaluation, but rather the thing done is the focus."[3]

Oftentimes the ADD/HD child does not seem to express guilt or remorse over being unable to perform in a prescribed manner, since without the association of value or meaning, he truly does not retain the information or instructions. The "mind" does not register that the information or request is worth retaining and is not nearly as interesting as whatever is going on in the child's head.

Similarly, Fossum and Mason say in their book *Facing Shame*, "While guilt is a painful feeling of regret and responsibility for one's actions, shame is a painful feeling about oneself as a person."[4] When the child fully realizes that he cannot perform in a way that is expected of him, the child internalizes that this will affect the way that he will be loved and accepted. The negative impacts are increased when it is also communicated that the child should be able to do those things and are making some kind of oppositionary choice. To the

---

2 Wikipedia: http://en.wikipedia.org/wiki/Shame#cite_note-4

3 ^ Lewis, Helen B. (1971), *Shame and guilt in neurosis*, International University Press, New York, ISBN 0-8236-8307-9

4 ^ Fossum, Merle A.; Mason, Marilyn J. (1986), *Facing Shame: Families in Recovery*, W.W. Norton, p. 5, ISBN 0-393-30581-3

outsider it appears at times as if the child is willingly disobeying when they are actually experiencing *"unwilling willing disobedience."*

Following this line of reasoning, psychiatrist Judith Lewis Herman concludes, "Shame is an acutely self-conscious state in which the self is 'split,' imagining the self in the eyes of the other; by contrast, in guilt the self is unified."[5] If there truly is a splitting of self within the mind of the ADD/HD individual, then it plays out in highly successful behavior with a self-abusive shadow side, or as highly dysfunctional behavior with tons of unrealized potential that keeps showing up enough to keep people committed to the cause of helping him.

Shame plays out in these children because they feel as though they have to hide their differences. They become confused with their version of how they see themselves in the world and how others communicate to them that they are seen in the world. This is one of the major contributors to the significant number of ADD/HD individuals who end up with addictions such as alcohol or drugs or become "rage-aholics" or workaholics. They can easily become addicted to computer games or to other things where they thrive and, in the process, avoid situations where they feel unable to fit in or do it the "right" way.

Fear

The factors of anxiety, isolation, shame and fear can play out in many different ways. In order to make a difference in the life of the ADD/HD child, it is necessary to understand that all of the aforementioned issues are playing out in varying degrees. Depending on the personality, upbringing, and support or lack thereof of the individual, these factors will play out differently. Let us first examine how and why they are caused. Instead of giving specific examples for each, the following example alone will be used to highlight anxiety, isolation, shame, and fear.

Let us call our child Chris. Between the ages of three and four, Chris begins to realize that he is different from the other children around him. He is even different from the expectations that his parents have of him. He does not seem to respond the way they expect him to respond. They may question his

---

5 ^ Herman, Judith Lewis (2007), "Shattered Shame States and their Repair", *The John Bowlby Memorial Lecture*

responses. They may question why he is not as "happy" as he should be about some experience. He feels happy, but he is not as outwardly expressive as expected. He tends to have a harder time sleeping and is often wound up to the point that he fidgets. His sense of curiosity is overwhelming. He understands more than he has developed the vocabulary to express and, when not being driven by all this energy, he can be quite content to be lost in his own little world. It is starting to dawn on our little Chris how different he is, although he may be well on the way to age five before he really begins to put it all together. Let us not forget that Chris is an extremely bright and sensitive child—not sensitive to criticism (though he may be), but sensitive to energy. By the time Chris moves from four to five, he definitely notices any anxiety within the household. Chris has also had more and more interaction with other children and sees the differences between them and him. Though he may not quite be sure yet that they are bad, these differences sure do not look good.

Chris then begins developing the intellectual emotional body. He knows that the people around him are starting to become concerned and he definitely does not want to be different in a bad way. He starts to feel like he has something he needs to keep hidden, something he must learn to control. His need to be active is now being called hyperactive and his lack of emotions are being referred to as odd, even though he does have emotions and they seem wild and uncontrolled when they come. He might have even heard himself discussed as a problem or overheard that he might need to go see a doctor to see what is wrong with him. Depending on when he begins school or preschool, these issues become more pronounced. By this point, Chris has learned shame and fear. The more he interacts with a world where he does not fit in, the more Chris also starts dealing with anxiety, the anxiety that he is going to do something which will make him stand out in a bad way. He begins to fear that his parents will stop loving him. He wonders why he is such a "bad" child and the more he feels like no one understands him, the more he feels isolated. He feels that no one really understands what is going on inside of him and if they knew, then they would really stop loving him.

Our little Chris, depending on the parents, the school system, and other environmental factors, finally comes to the inevitable conclusion that he is defective, disabled, undesirable, and even unlovable. There are many paths that Chris can take with that information, but they all unfold from the misconception that he is a problem and is somehow bad or wrong.

If you think that telling the child you love him will make him feel lovable, you will find that you are wrong more often than not. I have worked with many young adults and children whose parents tell them that they love them. However, because they are contending with all these other factors and fears, they still feel that they are broken or unlovable. I hear over and over again: "Do not tell my parents about how bad I am because they will not love me anymore." How can you be lovable when everyone has convinced you that you are defective and broken? To compound the issue, these other people do not understand what is going on inside of the ADD/HD child because not even they understand it. So how do you help them?

Challenges of Language

Words have meaning; they can shape and influence different realities, experiences, and even the way someone views themselves, others, and the world. Everything about communication, including context, tone, the energy with which things are said, and what actions surround the words, plays into how things are interpreted. Because communication is a two-way street, it is not only how things are said but also how they are heard that matter. ADD/HD children often do not process subtlety well. They can be quite literal because they have so much going on inside their heads early on, that some kinds of humor can be beyond their grasp. However, because they are sensitive to the energy with which things are conveyed, one must not only be careful of what one is saying but also how one is saying it and with what energies.

Another important factor at play here is if you are saying one thing but meaning another, they often will pick up on the dichotomy. The following story portrays this concept. A young ADD/HD man with whom I was working with, did not believe his mother when she said, after reading my first "Managing The Gift" book, that he did not have a disability but had a diff-ability. However, when I told him the same thing he believed me. At first I wanted to just chalk it up to the dismissal of his mother's words because they came from his mother. Upon speaking with his mother though, I realized that he didn't believe it when she said it because *she* didn't believe it when she said it. When we talked it out more and she could embrace the concept better, he started believing that she *did* believe that he was not disabled. Therefore, if you do not understand how ADD/HD can be a gift; if you do not see how these children do not have a disability but they simply learn and process information and experiences differently; if you do not understand how it is an evolutionary process and are unwilling to accept that as much, if not more, of the problems being experienced by your child are the result of being an ADD/HD child in a non-ADD/HD world, then do not try to convince him of it.

Don't lie to your child, even if it is just to be kind. Sooner or later, they will figure out that you are not being truthful with them. Of course, I am not advocating being cruel here, just honest. I worked with one child who struggled with understanding whether or not she was disabled. She did not believe her parents when they said that she might have some challenges but that she certainly was not disabled. When I asked her why she didn't believe her parents she listed off other areas where she did not think they had been honest with her. She provided an example about her physical appearance. She was overweight but not obese, but when asked what they thought about her weight, her parents told her she was fine. She wanted to believe them, but between the cruel things that other kids said to her and what the media role models as a normal size for someone her age, plus her finding she was overweight when she looked up and found an age, height, & weight proportionality chart, she simply could not!

During the process of working with her, she actually went through a growth spurt and slimmed down to a weight proportional to her height. However, instead of her parents addressing her concern as real when it was an issue for her, they allowed their own biases and fears to get in the way and just kept telling her she was fine. This was an opportunity to work with their daughter to develop some action and consequences thought processes. They could have posed questions such as, "What do you eat? Do you exercise? What other things are you doing or not doing that might affect your body?" They could have even explored the growth spurt concept by having her research it. She was interested enough in the subject that they could have utilized it as a wonderful opportunity to engage her "mind". Besides all that, as she so eloquently put it to me in her eleventh year of age, "I don't trust what my parents say because when I was fat, they didn't want me to be fat, so they just kept telling me that I wasn't fat. So now that they tell me that I am not really disabled, why should I believe them? Especially when I have been diagnosed with ADD and everyone knows ADD is a disability." After discussing why I felt that "what everyone knows" does not mean that they are right and allowed her to debate the issue with me, she decided that she only had a disability if she let people give one to her.

Helping Your Child with Anxiety, Isolation, Shame, and Fear

1. Begin talking to your child at an early age about how differences are not only acceptable, but that they are a good thing.

2. As you see your child struggle with emotions, explain how people deal with emotions differently and try to help them understand how the emotional body works.

3. Figure out, as best you can, how all the child's different bodies work and begin working with your child to understand the process.

4. Avoid judgmental and/or comparison comments, even if they are in your child's favor.

5. When your child is confronted with "better than/worse than" comments, work with him to understand that being better at something does not indicate that the person is better, just better at a specific activity or task and that we all have things at which we are better.

6. When you have to use ADD/HD terms, always use words like "diff-ability", not disability. Stress to your child that they learn and feel differently and that even his "energy levels" are different. Promote the truth that all of these things are perfectly natural; they just do not occur as often, which is why one meets fewer people with them.

7. Always refer to ADD/HD as a gift and help your child understand that it is a gift.

8. Listen carefully. Be aware of where your child is getting negative feedback about who he is. Do not be afraid to stand up for your child, especially about issues to do with the school system.

9. Many things can exacerbate some of the normal differences of the ADD/HD impacted child. These need to be addressed before some of the other recommendations will really begin to help. These things include diet, use of supplements, monitoring the environment, and use of meditating and centering techniques. (See chapter on supporting cast)

10. Never let anyone bully you or your child into using medications. Make sure you have fully exhausted and truly utilized a holistic approach to help your child embrace his gifts.

11. Be willing to stretch your comfort zones and utilize resources other than those with which you may be familiar. Remember that it is your child's well-being at stake, so stretch and do it for him.

Parenting is loving, nurturing, and preparing your children for the world and helping them become the best THEM they can be. You can shape your child, like one can shape a piece of clay; however, no more than you can make the clay a piece of glass, can you make your child what they are not. They are not you, nor are they here to bear the burden of becoming who you could not become, to finish carrying on your dreams, or to be your version of who you wanted to be as a child.

Discover the unique and special individual your child is. Just because you liked or disliked something does not mean that he will. Just because you could or could not do something does not mean he can or cannot. Because you wanted or avoided certain paths or ways of being in the world does not mean he will. Life is all the more difficult when a child is physically like a mini-me of one of the parents or some other close relative because then he will get pushed to be emotionally, energetically, and intellectually like them.

Instill in your child to accept and love himself for who he is; help your child to make the most out of and persevere through their struggles; help him recognize his value and worth; teach the ADD/HD children *how* to think, not *what* to think. These are the things that will help your child most maximize his potential and live a happy life. Is that not what every parent wants for their child?

CHAPTER 4

LEARNING

Hooked on Learning

IN THIS SECTION, we will address the things that can help support ADD/
HD children, facilitate their educational experience and tap into their love
of learning. We will go through each of the areas of your child's life, cor-
responding with the areas outlined in the review section, plus add the social
component.

There are some important points to keep in mind when teaching ADD/
HD children. They love to learn, are inherently curious and usually by a young
age have created a rich inner landscape, have strongly developed imaginations
and assignment of what is of value to them and what is not. Let's explore these
characteristics more deeply.

Assignment of Value

What we decide we value throughout our lifetime changes. We base our
decisions on our experiences, along with a plethora of other factors, some of
which are easily understandable to ourselves and explainable to others and some
are not and many are never even thought about, as to why we value what we
value, unless we are asked.

Throughout our lifetime, playing in the background is some constant level of us being who we are, that also determines what we value in our life. Are we drawn more to music or sports, reading or cooking, very noisy experiences or very quiet ones?

Of course, our role models, our experiences, our place in the world and the expectations of us can greatly impact how and if we pursue what we value but it doesn't change that we value it. Maybe we value music because it draws and touches us in ways we do understand or cannot explain. We may even feel that we are incomplete without it. However, factors outside ourselves such as coming from a family that loves and supports music versus one that sees it as a hobby or even worse a waste of time and money, effects how we play it out. Aspects of who we are, shy or outgoing, musically gifted with an instrument or not, born with perfect pitch or sound like a cat in heat when we sing, also contribute to how we incorporate music in our lives. Does it become our career, whether that is by being a professional musician, singer, songwriter or as a music teacher? Do we become a conductor or just a collector, who surrounds ourselves with music? The role music plays in our life will be determined not only by how much we value it but by how much we value ourselves.

For the greater population, our need to fit in, belong, be loved and accepted allows us to be manipulated away from assigning the time, energy and priority to the things we value, if they are not perceived as practical, desirable or achievable by our tribe. We allow ourselves to spend the majority of our time, energy and focus on what other people determine as valuable, even when we don't get or understand why it is valuable to us or even in general. This may have been accomplished through emotional blackmail, physical intimidation, playing on fears, the good old-fashioned punishment and reward system of parenting and educating and most likely a combination of the above.

To a great extent the ADD/HD population seems to respond far less to others trying to manipulate them into spending time, energy and focus on things which they have not found value in, are not interested by or found the worth of. I address this more in the *"unwilling willing disobedience"* section. However, in the end the thing to remember here is, that unless this child finds value, worth or interest in, what you are asking them, on a consistent basis for a prolong period of time, not only can you not make them learn, do or remember it, they can't make themselves either. This is part of the evolutionary upgrade, whether we like it or not.

Mindless Memorization

The ADD/HD mind is like a sponge, always looking to soak up something new. The problem occurs when the mind begins to decide what it believes has meaning, purpose, value or interest and what does not. Memorization for the fact of memorization with no understandable reason almost seems to be beyond the ADD/HD mind. The ADD/HD mind can become a well of what might appear as useless or unimportant information to the outside world because what the mind remembers was of interest or fascinating to that person with ADD/HD. So often the push for mindless and what appears to be pointless memorization in our current educational model takes what should be a joyful and enthusiastic experience and turns it into a negative, disempowering, high-anxiety experience for your child. The children and adults around your child can often end up with a very convoluted concept of his abilities and potentials.

The repetition style of learning is also another way in which the ADD/HD mind gets turned against traditional learning. Because the ADD/HD mind gets bored easily, if it has made the decision that something is interesting enough to undertake then your child must be kept moving through the process of learning it as thoroughly as he can. So when he knows he can add and adds five or six problems in a row successfully, he looses all interest in adding up ten more unless there is something more challenging about it. Proving to someone else you know the concept is not part of the mind's nature. If it is part of your child's nature to please people, or if a fear of rejection or reprimand makes him want to prove it, then the mind and your child go into a tug of war which creates frustration. The task is simply not challenging enough to keep the mind engaged, no matter how important it is to your child emotionally.

Curiosity

Hand in hand with loving to learn is the curiosity factor. The problem with ADD/HD learners is that often, their curiosity leads them to a place that they are not content to leave until their curiosity is satiated. Remember, it is a myth that these kids can not focus; they either hyper-focus or multi-task. Therefore, when their curiosity is engaged, they want to hyper-focus and when what is being presented does not interest them, they multi-task. Repetition and the ensuing boredom is the death knoll to their ability to pay attention. The greatest distraction from but also supporter of their curiosity is the imagination.

Imagination

Early in the development process the ADD/HD child is soaking up every kind of experience and piece of information he can get his hands on. Your child is filling up his brain with stuff from which he can launch his own inner landscape and imagination. The more pieces your child has in place and the more he begins to create, co-create and re-create within his own head, the harder it is to get him to engage with outside experiences and information, which is not deemed worthy. This is one of the situations where critical thinking skills and interactive dialogue teaching methods are most effective in assisting your child to see a reason or purpose for really focusing on what you are trying to teach him. Of course, if what you are trying to teach has no real meaning or value in his life, good luck. This is why sometimes social morays, traditions and things we do just to please someone else seem to go right over the ADD/HD head.

The next step is to determine into which of the ADD/HD sub-categories your child falls to discover the most effective methods for teaching your child. Then it is important to figure out with which learning and processing styles your child most identifies to create an effective educational plan.

Helping Your Child Learn by "Painting Their Portrait"

The better you understand your child from a number of different perspectives, the easier it is to support, guide and parent him as well as create a teaching game plan that should be used with him. I have often been told by educators that any child would benefit from this approach in creating educational plans, but with the ADD/HD child it is imperative if you would like your child to reach his full potential and do so medication free.

The parent cannot expect that his child's teacher is going to be able to immediately know all the different aspects of the child that can help set up an education plan that will help the child succeed. The parent, who has the history with the child, needs to be able to work with these insights to help the teacher. After all, in most cases the teacher has just met the child and has anywhere from twenty to thirty other children about whom they also need to learn.

Before the school year starts, make sure you have updated the overall picture of your child of who they are and how they function. As children grow, expand and discover more of who they are and also are changed by the world, you want to be constantly updating the picture you have painted of your child to reflect these changes. This will help you present an accurate portrait of your child to a teacher to best support them in the process of helping your child learn.

Some of the results of this will not change or will change very little from year to year. Highlight the applicable suggestions and add to them your insights and experiences regarding what works and what does not work for your child, and give it, along with a copy of this book, to everyone who is going to be working with your child in any significant way. If your child is on an educational plan of some kind, make sure these things are included in it. Then it is your job to follow up, making sure that everything to best assist your child is being done. Waiting for the teacher to come to know your child or for your child to adjust to a new teacher along with a new set of rules, routines, and classmates is setting your child up for failure.

What Is Their Canvas?

Our intellectual level was designed to reason, to envision and to analyze. It was created to be both a recorder and a communicator of our human experience. It is both the master and servant to our physical level, our emotional level and our spiritual level.

First, how do we think? I am going to break it down into categories that I will call *styles*. There are learning, processing, and thinking styles. When we get to the ADD/HD impact, our understanding of these styles will help us differentiate between the challenges brought about by ADD/HD and environmental issues that are being blamed on ADD/HD. Here is an overview of the impacts/shifts level by level drawn from *Managing The Gift: Alternative Approaches For Attention Deficit Disorder.*

Learning Styles

There have been many books written on styles of learning, covering a multitude of combinations and tangential learning styles. For our purposes, we will look at three basic learning styles: *auditory*, *visual* and *kinesthetic*. Of course, there are combinations of the three.

Auditory Learning

Auditory learning is the kind of learning style where hearing is the easiest and most efficient way for someone to understand or grasp a concept. When people with this learning style become quiet, pay attention and listen, they will learn or understand what is being taught. You might identify this type by observing them when they are trying to understand something difficult. It is not unusual for them to close their eyes, even tilt their head as if they are trying to tune their ear in to hear the person teaching and tune out everything else around them. If you give auditory learners directions, they will listen intently, repeat them back to you and then go. If you change anything in the directions after the auditory learner repeats them to you, they will assimilate the changes and most likely repeat the whole thing over again with the corrected information. Hearing themselves say it commits the information to memory.

Visual Learning

Visual learning involves seeing something in order to best comprehend it. Visual learners see it on the blackboard or read it in a book or even write it down. These learners may be copious note-takers, not only jotting down what is written on the board but also for whatever the teacher says. They may never actually read the notes because the act of committing it to paper is enough. If you give these learners directions, they will write them down and may even draw a map. When they drive, they may never look at the directions because seeing them written down was enough.

Kinesthetic Learning

Kinesthetic learners learn by doing and interacting. If you can involve them in the process, they will understand. Kinesthetic learning is linked to kinetics, the energy of movement. If there is movement involved, kinesthetic learners do better, even if the movement is yours. If you show them how to do something by doing it, it is more helpful than telling them, giving them something to read about it or writing it on the board. If you give these children directions, they are likely to be tracing the movements in midair or on a table. Their hands may be making left and right motions or any other gestures that help commit the information to memory.

In my years in corporate America, I often held training or training manager positions. I learned that the best way to do standard training was the following:

- Have them read about what you are getting ready to teach them

- Then tell them what you are going to tell them

- Tell them

- Show them

- Then tell them what you told them

You accomplish this by:

- Having them tell you what you told them

- Then show you what you showed them

- The ultimate step in the process is to observe them teaching someone else

Depending on what you are teaching, the process is sometimes easy, but other times it must become far more creative. This is an extremely efficient teaching method as it incorporates all three learning styles. Most people have a primary and secondary learning style. Although they both work at some level, one will always be more effective. I will not say that success is ensured with this training style, but the success rate is high. The big factor "x" in these scenarios has nothing to do with ability. It is usually about desire. People who want to learn something, consciously or unconsciously, will lead you to the learning style they need—if you let them. They may ask questions, ask for something to read or ask you to demonstrate and work with them. If the chore of learning becomes too difficult or too cumbersome, they will lose interest.

Processing Styles

The two basic styles of processing are *internal* and *external*. These styles have nothing to do with personality or whether the person is outgoing and extroverted or shy and introverted, and unfortunately, people often automatically assume they go hand-in-hand. Because I have a very outgoing personality, people often assume that I process things externally whereas a former partner of mine kept more to himself and therefore people assumed that he had an internal processing style. However, it was just the reverse! In fact, we were at a conference a few years ago and one of the other people there was studying iridology, the science of receiving information about people through the study of their eyes. She asked if she could look into our eyes and tell us what she saw. On other occasions and throughout the four days of the conference, she had spent a fair amount of social time with us. She first looked into my eyes and then without saying anything called my partner over, looked into his eyes and then looked at both of us again. She then told us, with a fair amount of surprise in her voice, that I was the introvert and my partner was the extrovert. We confirmed her information, since we had already figured that out. So, what do I mean when I talk about internal and external when it comes to processing styles?

External

A child with an *external* processing style likes to think through things by getting whatever they are processing outside of themselves. In other words, they need to talk it through with someone else to figure out what they are thinking and feeling about something. The funny thing is that it is not unusual for the other person not to say anything at all! It is simply the act of processing or working through something aloud that helps external processors. Sometimes they want input and other times they just need to get it out. When they have reached some kind of conclusion which is acceptable and manageable in their own mind, they are open to receiving input. If you try to give them input too quickly, it will distract them from their own processes and they will likely either snap at you or shut down.

External processors become stuck in their head and need to literally "get out of their head" so they can sort through something. By giving them more or new information, they end up back in their head with the information and are in danger of being stuck again. This is especially true of people who have a tendency to be caught in thought loops. A thought loop is an idea or set of ideas to which one keeps returning. It seems impossible to break the loop. One of the more challenging aspects of the external processing style is that it takes them a very long time (if it ever does happen) to figure out and be able to ask the person with whom they are processing to give them what they need. This is because they do not understand what it is that they need. Oftentimes, the person dealing with an external processor will try to "fix" the problems instead of just hearing them out. This is not helpful until external processors get to a point where they are specifically asking for feedback. In addition, children with this processing style can contradict themselves many times before finally coming to the point of resolution, creating even more confusion for the listener.

Internal

Children, whose processing style is *internal,* process things by going within themselves to understand that about which they are unresolved. The two kinds of internal processing are *conscious* and *unconscious.* Conscious internal processing involves the child working through it within his own head, weighing pros and cons, and then coming to some kind of decision or conclusion. The child with the unconscious style of internal processing may or may not weigh pros and cons, but they do not consciously come to a conclusion or a decision. It is as if they forget about it or put it out of their mind and then suddenly they "know" how they feel about something; they have decided or reached a definite conclusion.

This does not mean the child with an internal processing pattern does not get additional information or consult other people, but the real work happens within his mind. Sometimes he might be asking questions or steering conversations in certain directions with no concept as to why. The child is just gathering information.

Recharging Styles

There are two kinds of recharging styles, *introverted* and *extroverted*. The first thing to remember when understanding how these styles function and how to best work with them is that they have nothing to do with whether the child is outgoing or not. They indicate whether the child needs solitude or time around other people to refuel themselves. An introverted child can be quite outgoing, but if not given regular intervals of solitary activity or alone time, they become overwhelmed and will begin to act out or meltdown. Extroverted children at times may be quiet and observant and appear to be non-participatory, yet if they do not get regular time where they are around other people, whether just a couple of people or a whole group, they get out of sorts and cranky. One child may simply draw energy from being with others, yet another would become drained spending too much time around other people, or large groups of people. Therefore, when painting the portrait of your child, pay attention to whether or not the child's amount of connected time or alone time seems to be linked to any meltdowns or bad behaviors he may play out. Understanding your child's recharging style helps you build into the child's life what the child needs, even when he does not understand it or know how to ask for it.

Looking at your child with both of the perspectives in mind of how they recharge and process, you might discover that you have an outgoing extrovert who is an internal processor or that you have a child who tends to be a soft spoken introvert who actually needs to process in an external way.

Thinking Styles

The two main styles of thinking are *analytical* and *abstract*. These are often associated with masculine/yang and feminine/yin energy. This is not wholly incorrect, but it does not have anything to do with being male or female. However, the connection is often what pushes us to believe that males are better in math and science and females in the arts and languages. This conditioning pushes children of both sexes to nurture the subjects positively associated with their particular gender and ignore or be discouraged from exploring what we associate with the opposite gender qualities and characteristics. In working with ADD/HD children and adults, I have actually discovered a third thinking style, which I have called spiral which seems to kick in when they are in a problem solving/learning mode.

Analytical

Analytical thinking is sequential in nature. It is also associated with logical thinking. It is left brain thinking and deals well with things that fall into some kind of orderly or discernable pattern. It is a thinking style that is very action-oriented. It tries to make everything orderly, practical and logical. The focus tends to be quite solution-oriented, with goals tending towards those things that are simple, quick and efficient. Analytical thinking is definitely a style that is much more comfortable with a "black and white" reality. It will often reject that which has not or can not be proven.

Abstract

Abstract thinking is a style geared towards probabilities and possibilities as much as facts. This right brain thinking pairs things together which may have no logical connections and are more conceptual in nature. Abstract thinkers are much more willing to follow hunches and see where these hunches will take them rather than being content with what the facts indicate. Creative and inventive, their road to a solution may be hard, if not impossible, to follow. This does not make it any less likely to be correct, just harder to explain. They are less interested in the "what" of a situation and more interested in the "why." It is not the surface "why" they are interested in but the deeper "why."

Spiral

After spending a great deal of time within the ADD/HD population and challenging these gifted individuals, I began to notice a new pattern emerging in their thinking style. Rather than having an analytic or abstract thinking style, which one might picture as a straight line, they think in a way that would more resemble an ever-widening spiral staircase.

Truly bright, non-ADD/HD people in the past who developed the ability to think and process from both their left and right brains, shifting as required, still thought in a pattern that looked more angular in nature. Spiral thinking is another of those evolutionary steps where the process has blended into a new thought style, which increases the potential number of solutions when analyzing a problem. Spiral thinking is synergetic in nature because the thoughts are actually happening in a way that is simultaneous in nature and feed off of each other. Not all ADD/HD children have this thinking style but rather some have a highly developed switching station where they move from abstract to analytical in the blink of an eye. The true spiral thinker would begin with whatever thought process came most naturally to them and then would move into simultaneously examining the issue from both analytic (left brain) thinking and abstract (right brain) thinking perspectives. Depending on how much they are verbalizing what is going on, it may appear as if they are alternating styles when in actuality it is happening synergistically.

Star Trek fans will recognize the image of the chess board which exists on separate planes, where one must look at all three planes of the chess board in order to make a decision on where to move. The move from a one dimensional chess board where we have a finite set of considerations and ways to strategize, problem solve and play out future possibilities to a three level chess board where things are looked at in a more multi-dimensional way is one of the better analogies, though still inadequate, about the difference between how the ADD/HD versus the non-ADD/HD brain takes in, processes, integrates and then builds upon incoming information.

These individuals, when interested, focused, engaged and motivated, seem to be traveling in this multi-dimensional, spiral pattern, which allows them to come up with ideas, thoughts, solutions and questions (ESPECIALLY questions) that appear to come out of nowhere and nobody ever thought to ask before. Like the three dimensional chessboard, they come at it from angles that hitherto we would not have come from or even considered as possible. Also because they tend to be highly intuitive in nature, this is also a strong factor which plays within their thinking style. Like three strands of a braid, the ability to entwine abstract, analytical and intuitive thoughts have created a very powerful and increased access to more of the human potential. That is how these brains played off of each other and created the advancements of the twentieth century. To witness this phenomenon, however, one must have them interested and engaged. One must also listen to the questions they ask more than the responses they give and ferret out from where the questions came.

So often, if the individual listening can't immediately see the validity of the question, the person assumes that the child's mind is just wandering disconnectedly from the conversation. Only with patience, supportive energies, an open mind and good questions can they start to see where some of the questions came from and that they are not irrelevant at all. Remember, if the person is an external processor, they will take the listener around the barn a couple of times before the listener can make sense of what is being said. However, if the listener shuts the child down by interrupting or trying to adjust something that has been said before the child is finished speaking, he will stop taking the risk of sharing and may just turn all questions and thought processes inward. It can also negatively affect how the child perceives or feels about himself.

Information Handling

There are two groups in this category with each group having two different primary ways of interacting in the world. The first group has to do with how they best *attach* to the information and the second is how they *work* with that information.

Attaching to a piece of information comes through one of two ways: *passionate* or *rational perspectives*. We all have experienced having someone tell us something that we couldn't really connect with, we might understand it but we don't attach to it. Attaching is interacting, owning, and making it yours which is a crucial key to engaging the ADD/HD brain when you want it to learn, work with or even remember something you are sharing. The *passionate* child initially gets excited about the idea, concept or task and then once "hooked" will go into that hyper-focused place where he can then absorb and work with the knowledge. The *rational* child needs it to make sense to him; he has to understand logically where the information fits into his view of self and the world.

In working with information, there are also two styles: *direct* and *manipulate*. Children with the *direct* style prefer to take the information head on and work with it on two levels at the beginning. At first, they seek to understand it and how it applies to their world. Then, they communicate or teach that information. In the process of sharing, they will often move into the "how to reshape and change it" mode. However, to get them to really take it in and own it the door way to accomplishing that is marked: direct.

On the other hand, *manipulators* take the information, once they have decided the information or task is interesting or of value to them and immediately begin reworking it even while they are even still trying to understand it. Their first urge is to see how they can improve it, shift it, change it, and work with it in different ways. At some point, it is likely they will want to teach it, but their first stop is to play with the ideas, information, and/or tasks, that have caught their attention.

Creating The Portrait

The portrait is not meant to be just labels but rather to be utilized as a guide through which you can put together better ways to communicate with and for your child, as well as create a better educational plan for your child.

The following questions are broken into two categories. The first category represents the questions that apply to any person. Through understanding these questions, the individual has better self-awareness and can better express his needs in order to best take in and process not only information but also life as a whole. Doing this first part for any child can help facilitate a better understanding of how to help, support and educate that child. The second category is specifically designed to aid the ADD/HD child.

Your Child's Style

1. Does the child need alone time/solitary activity to cope? (Introvert)

2. Does the child need one on one or group time to cope? (Extrovert)

3. Does the child need to get inward thoughts/information outside of themselves and talk it out, without interruption, to obtain clarity regarding whether or not they understand it, and if not, what is it they need in order to get clarity? (External Processor)

4. Do you need to give the child the information, send them off to do something else, preferably repetitive or brainless, and then check back in with the child later? (Internal processor)

5. Does the child get excited when becoming interested in something new and immediately try to shift, change or improve it in someway? (Passionate)

6. When becoming interested in something, does the child tend to analyze it and question you in a manner that seems to come out more like accusations, almost as if they are testing you? (Direct)

ADD/HD Intellectual Patterns

1. When expressing themselves, do their thoughts come out as a stream of consciousness but seem to have some relationship among themselves but seem to be never ending? (DSL)

2. When expressing thoughts, do they interrupt themselves with things that seem completely unrelated and to come out of nowhere? (Pulse)

3. When expressing thoughts, do they follow a thought process to a place where either they have lost interest or have satisfactorily (for them) figured out where they were going, then jump to thoughts that are sometimes related and sometimes completely non sequitur? (Spaghetti)

ADD/HD Energy Patterns

1. Does your child have high energy but it is pretty consistent while doing things that simulate physical activity, such as riding around in a car. Does he seem to struggle with writing clearly or reading? (Steady)

2. Does your child seem to have very erratic energy patterns? Can he be hypnotized by TV & computer games AND gets almost violent or melts down when suddenly shaken out of either activity? Does he struggle with writing clearly and can't sit still for the longer periods of time necessary to really get into reading? (Pulse)

3. Does your child seem to have both of the above patterns occurring at different times? Watch for a rhythm or a pattern of moving from one to another. (Crescendo)

Once the chart is filled out, then you start to bring together the pieces to complete the portrait. Below I have the strategies and insights for the ADD/HD-based qualities as well as the groupings of thought, attachment and processing style. Merging these last two answers together on the chart help round out the program you are creating.

Thought, Attachment, and Processing Styles

Although I went over five categories for you to assess your child on: Recharging, Learning, Thought, Attachment, and Processing, I only chose the last three for the chart to both keep it simple and it provided the best way to utilize the information when utilizing or giving insights about how to best work with your child. Ideal teaching is always done in multiple learning formats and knowing whether your child needs alone time or connected time to recharge seemed to be easy add-ons.

PASSIONATE

EXTERNAL-DIRECT	INTERNAL-DIRECT
• This child needs very directive information; it must engage a current passion or capture the imagination.	• This child needs very directive information; it must engage a current passion or capture the imagination.
• Give the child actions to take to engage him more fully. This child will not do subtle well.	• You should give the child actions to take to engage him more fully. This child will not do subtle well.
• Be direct, engage the heart and give him a sense of responsibility and actions to take.	• Be direct, engage the heart and give him a sense of responsibility and actions to take.
• Get the child into a place where he has to explain, demonstrate and teach it.	• You give this child the information/task and ask him to be inventive with it.
• Have this child talk out what he is thinking or feeling about what you have asked him to do or process.	• Let the child take the information and process it and have him give you a list of questions, thoughts or ways to make it better or do it differently.

EXTERNAL-MANIPULATIVE	INTERNAL-MANIPULATIVE
• This child needs to be led to the conclusions; a case needs to be built that will make obvious the connection.	• Get this child excited about the information or task, giving him just enough information to grasp its basic concepts.
• The information/task must be presented in a way that engages a current passion or captures the child's imagination.	• Then send the child away to come up with better ways to do it, different ways to apply it, a deadline, plus an opportunity to present it.
• Also, give the child the opportunity to play out different scenarios. Let him interact with the information until he takes ownership for it.	• If the child is more outgoing/extroverted in nature, then have him present it to the class or the group.
• To help the child engage with the information/task, have him immediately go into problem-solving mode.	• If the child is more outgoing/introverted in nature, then you may want him to present it to a small group.
• Have the child talk through how he is going to do it or what the information means to him.	• If the child is quieter (whether extroverted or introverted) in nature, have the child present it to an adult with whom he trusts and feels comfortable.
• Give the child some ways to recreate it but have him talk it through before implementation.	

RATIONAL

EXTERNAL-DIRECT	INTERNAL-DIRECT
• This child needs to understand where this information or task fits into his world and why it makes sense for him to acquire the ability to work with or understand the information.	• This child needs to understand the logic or rationale behind the task or why the information needs to be learned.
• Show the child the logic behind the information being presented and send the child away with a deadline to come up with different ways to teach it.	• Spell it out to this child and challenge him regarding how to take action, apply and even share the information.
• If the child is more outgoing, have the child teach the class (after you have made sure the child truly understands it).	• Give this child straightforward examples and analogies.
• If the child is outgoing/introverted in nature, then you may want the child to teach it to a small group.	• Then send the child away to come up with some of his own.
• If the child is quieter in nature, have him teach it back to you or observe him teach it to one other person.	• Challenge the child to teach it back to you in a different way than you taught it to him.
EXTERNAL-MANIPULATIVE	INTERNAL-MANIPULATIVE
• This child needs to be led to the logic of the information/task through building on logic that is already in place.	• Show this child where this information or task fits into his world and why it makes sense for him to acquire the ability to work with or understand the information.
• Attach it to a goal that he wants to have.	• Show the child the logic behind the information being presented and send the child away with a deadline to come up with different ways to work with the information or different applications for the task.
• Help the child think of different ways that the information can be utilized.	• If the child is more outgoing/extroverted, have him teach the class (after you have made sure the child truly understands it).
• Engage the child in the where and the how that the information or task could be shifted.	• If the child is outgoing/introverted in nature, then you may want the child to present it to a small group.
• Engage him in discussions that appear non-related as example and analogies; then send the child away to figure out why they do relate.	• If the child is quieter (whether extroverted or introverted) in nature, have the child teach it back to you or observe the child teach it to one other person.

CHAPTER 5

SUPPORTING AND GUIDING

SUPPORTING AND GUIDING your child are very different activities, but oftentimes as your child gets older they can become quite entwined. Supporting your child is holding your child up and helping her through life as she figures out how to navigate the world. This means helping her to do so in a way that allows her to be who she is and get what she wants in as joyful a way as possible. Guiding your child is pushing her out into the world and holding her accountable for what you have given her, and for what you have taught and shown her.

If too much support is given and not enough guidance, children either remain dependent or become recklessly independent during their teen years or early twenties. With too much support, they internalize that either you do not think they can do things on their own or even worse they truly aren't capable. Also, trying to guide them too quickly and forcing them toward a level of independence for which they may not yet be ready sets them up for failure. Therefore, as we review ways to best support and guide your child, I will most often delineate which of the two is in play.

When painting the picture of your child earlier, one of the things you were asked to discern was your child's processing and recharging styles. Is your child introverted or extroverted and is she an internal or an external processor? This is an important distinction to keep in mind when you are guiding your child. Do remember, though, to not fall into the trap of believing that if your child is outgoing, that she is automatically an external processor or an extrovert; likewise, if your child is quiet, she is not necessarily an internal processor or introvert. This processing style is simply how your child recharges so that she does not get overwhelmed or overloaded.

Transitions

Oftentimes, transitions from one environment to another are difficult for children with ADD/HD. Going from school to home tends to be high on the list of difficult transitions. One of the big reasons is the shift in structure. The challenge of working with ADD/HD individuals, children, and adults is that they need structure. However, if given too much structure, they become destructive or self-destructive because they feel claustrophobic; if not given enough structure, they cannot get off the launching pad. With just the right amount of structure they can fly. However, it is not a "one size fits all" structure. It is just as much about the kinds of structure as how much structure is provided.

Going from the environment of school to home often causes your child to meltdown or act out in any number of different ways. This is typically related to the great pressure and structure at school that is often incompatible with your child's needs. The more compatible the structure is where your child has been to where your child is going, plus the more aligned the places are to the structure your child needs, the easier the transition. These kinds of transitions can be seamless. Consistency is also key. Because ADD/HD children at an early age can start to have performance anxiety and feel like oddities, teaching them how to reduce undesirable outcomes is of essential importance. The fewer worries these children have regarding ridicule and blame, the more relaxed and "go with the flow" they are able to be. After-school meltdowns can happen for a number of different reasons:

1. Emotional drops

2. Physical energy overload

3. Built-up anxiety

4. Over stimulation from peers

5. Physical environment of the school itself

6. When and what they ate and drank.

Sometimes your child has spent all day trying to hold it together as they are swimming upstream in an environment which is inharmonious emotionally with them, or is even physically painful for them. The sooner you can help your child to identify when things started not feeling or being right, the quicker adjustments can be made to help alleviate the after-school meltdowns.

Introverted-Internal

If your child is introverted and an internal processor, then when she comes home allow her to engage in comforting solitary activities. Let her know that in a little bit you are going to ask how her day went, but do not put her on the spot immediately. She will likely just give you a one word answer that tells you how she is in this moment but not how her day went and won't want to discuss it further. Sometimes she will just say something along the lines of "I dunno know" because by asking her on the spot, often she truly does not know. If in the past you have determined that the issues leading to the meltdown seem to be more of a physical build up rather than something that happened at school, then direct your child to do something that will release the energy. Playing with a pet can be very helpful. If she has a *steady* energy pattern, then some *limited* time on the computer or TV, if it simulates motions, is an option when play is not. If you know that there is some emotional anxiety attached, then help her choose play activities or even chores which will allow for both a physical release of energy as well as a chance to talk about what is going on in her world, such as using a punching bag or raking leaves. Doing something physical with a trusted adult which allows her to communicate with that adult when she feels ready can be very helpful.

If your child's energy pattern is *pulse* or *pulse burst*, then escalating play is better such as going from walking to running to sprinting. Avoid computer and TV altogether until she has released the build up. Encourage roughhousing and things that have an element of unpredictability. Playing with you or an older, more mature playmate that can ensure that the play does not trigger a meltdown but helps supports the release.

Both kinds of introverts can do well with playing music as a release. Encourage them to try string, woodwind instruments or piano; instruments where the music is as much of an internalized experience as an outward performance. For manipulative types of children, encourage them to "create the music"; with directive types, encourage them to take a piece they know or have been practicing and play with it, finding a different way to perform it. Use art to help them draw or paint their experiences, especially if they are manipulative versus directive. If they are directive, they may move more towards sculpting. Have them create one piece of art of demonstrating how their day went and another showing how they wanted it to go.

Whether steady or pulse, before you send your child out to release the build up, let her know that when she is done, you want to hear about her day and how it could have gone better. Sometimes this might not even happen until bedtime, but remind her that you want to know. Structure this discussion so that your child gets the sense that she is allowed to stay up a little later by telling you, but if she is reticent to talk about it, then she goes right to bed. All of this has been supporting her. When your child shares where the day did not go well or how she wishes it had gone, then guide her to make connections regarding what she could have done differently in order to make it better in the future. Use this time to coach her on some of the techniques she has been given. Have her think about how, if these techniques had been used, the day would have gone differently. Tie it back to the actions/consequences model. For example, let's say your child had to do a time out because she acted out and you also find out that she ate some candy previous to acting out. If your child knows that candy makes her act that way, do not yell or punish; just point it out. Get her to think through whether having a treat that had negative consequences is better than having a treat which would have had no consequences. Give her these types of scenarios and let her think about them. If you are having this discussion at bedtime, then let her sleep on it and talk with her about it again in the morning.

Extroverted-Internal

The major difference between how to deal with the aforementioned types and extroverted-internal types, is to get these children involved with other children or some kind of group activity where they can refill themselves as they are processing internally. One might think that because of being surrounded by other children all day, extroverted-internal children would be overflowing with resource energies. However, if the environment was stressful or angst-ridden, it does not create the right kind of replenishment energy. They need to replenish by being with someone in a loving, low stress way to get back to a more balanced state and not become out of sorts and energetically tired.

Extroverted- External

If your child is *external-steady*, then find a rhythmic activity that the two of you can do together. During the activity, have her process her day with you. If the processing stops, then so does the activity. If your child is external and a *pulse*, find irregular activities where she can become as energetic as necessary but still maintain the conversation. If she is having a difficult time expressing a feeling that she had during the day, see if she can act or dance it out; associate it with some part of the activity that you are doing. With this type of child, you may have to allow the processing to take a backseat for a few minutes and then re-engage it.

Both kinds of extroverts often find release through playing music. Encourage them to utilize drums or percussion instruments, for with these instruments create a vibration that better supports a release of energies for these children. With pulse-direct children, let them play for release; allow them to play not for the sake of making music but rather so that they can express how they are feeling. With *pulse-manipulative* children, have them work with some guidelines of a known piece and improvise. Let the music be discordant in nature. With steady types of children, encourage more expression in flow. The music can still be loud or frustrated or angry, but have it follow a pattern. There will be more release in it for them. In art, have extroverts construct or build something; *pulse-direct* children (especially with a crescendo pattern) may need to build, build, build and then destroy it by knocking it over or tearing it up. Do not chastise this behavior because it is the release for them. *Pulse-manipulative* children may need to build it up, build it up, build it up and then take it apart and do it all over again in a cyclical nature. Do not try to tell them it was fine the way it was or discourage them from needing to do it all over again. *Steady-direct* children may create until they believe the project to be finished; whether it is finished in anyone else's eyes or not, they walk away and are done with it. Do not egg them on to complete. Remember, we are talking about things to do to help them transition from an over-stimulated, high-anxiety or physically under-stimulated environment to more of an even keel. The secret is the transition, not a finished product. *Steady-manipulative* children may have to walk away and go back several times before they are done and keep creating/recreating; do not encourage them to move on until they are ready. If you have time deadlines, then work breaks in that let them go back and forth a couple of times before they have to move on to something else.

Introverted-External

In this case, time alone or one on one with a safe person needs to be created during the processing. In the above situations, often times the more people there are that are involved when getting the energies balanced and in harmony, the better. However, with an introverted external processor, alone time and one on one time with a safe source is the key. That source, a parent or consistent caregiver, must be very careful to remain discerning and not become judgmental regarding how the day went. The caregiver must engage this child in earlier stages of guidance, going back and forth between guidance to support. Sometimes a stuffed animal, pet or imaginary friend is a good way for the child to start the conversation.

When moving from supporting to guiding, with the externals, you still need to get them to either talk to you or a trusted, responsible source about their thoughts and feelings, possibly even have them write about them, so that they can get whatever they are struggling with outside of themselves. A key word here is responsible source. If your ADD/HD child feels as though understanding and support comes from someone who may not have the ability, understanding or maturity needed to play that role, it doesn't matter. She will still follow that individual's guidance. That is one of the reasons why your child must have an adult who she can trust, that doesn't fear she will disappoint or that she doesn't feel judged or criticized by. An adult that is capable of high level, critical thinking based interaction. An adult that will empower your child to figure out and make decisions for herself, at the highest level she is capable of.

Out in the World

Play dates and other transitions can also be rough. The key to navigating these situations is often having the consistency of a close, feel-safe playmate or adult, one who can spot the early warning signs of meltdown and can prompt their child to utilize some calming and centering techniques. If your child has gone into either an emotional drop or a built-up, physically necessitated energy meltdown, then the only thing to do is separate her and let her play it out. Trying to stop it only exacerbates it; let it play out as safely as possible and then when she is sufficiently recovered, use it as a learning tool and make sure that the proper actions/consequences are in place.

Another key issue here is to address whether or not you have set your child up to fail. Ignoring the warning signs and not being consistent with what you expect from your child, and expecting her to function at a higher maturity level than that of which she is capable are all problems that can result in failure for her. If you do not keep up your end of the bargain, then you need to explain that to your child and teach her the consequences you brought on yourself for your choice of actions. When something like this *does* happen, make sure that your child's consequences are in alignment with the whole situation. Also, use this as a guidance opportunity that does not negate your own responsibility but shows your child that the more self-responsible she is, the less she will be negatively affected by other people's poor choices.

Dad knows that when Jenna, age six, eats foods that are highly processed and contain high fructose corn syrup, she becomes manic, unreasonable and will end up having a tantrum when the high wears off. Jenna knows that these foods are really not good for her but is young enough that she still wants them. She is very good at not eating them without asking, though. Dad and Jenna are at a family gathering where almost everything looks good to a six year old. Jenna keeps asking if she could please, please, please have some of whatever has just caught her eye. Dad did not bring "healthy goodies" and Jenna feels left out. Also, all the adults keep telling him that a little will not hurt. Besides, all the cousins are eating those foods and Jenna does not have any goodies of her own. First, Dad needs to take the responsibility of seeing if he and Jenna can find something that will act like a goodie that will not have the negative play outs that eating the other goodies will. If there are none, then Dad should guide Jenna and himself toward solving the problem by perhaps finding something else that can make Jenna feel like she has her own "goodie", even if it is not food. If Jenna does decide that she really, really wants one of the processed foods, then Dad should troubleshoot and figure out what is the least toxic choice and allow Jenna to have just a small amount of it. Dad should support Jenna while she is making the decision and maybe even come up with a way that minimizes the effect of the treat, such as giving her some fruit if she begins to act or feel out of sorts after ingesting the cookie and making sure she drinks plenty of water with the cookie.

Even though your child may seem too young for this level of involvement in decision-making, the sooner you guide your child the best you can, of course depending upon the severity of the choice your child wants to make, the better able your child will be to make decisions and hold fast when the consequence from the action shows up, whether good or bad.

Helping Them Fly

Completion of self-directed projects, adult-directed projects and staying on task all seem to be consistent struggles. Homework definitely falls into these categories as well. ADD/HD individuals of any age need just enough structure from which to fly. If not given enough, they never get off the ground; if given too much, they feel claustrophobic and destroy the structure. Determining the right amount of structure depends on the following factors.

If the answer is yes to any of the following questions, then provide your child with *less* structure:

1. Is this something that your child has chosen to undertake which has put them into hyper focus?

2. Is this something that has captured your child's interest in the moment?

3. Are they hyper-focused? If so, they may need help with time awareness.

If the answer is yes to any of the following questions, then provide your child with *more* structure:

1. Is this something you had to sell to your child?

2. Is this something that is interesting enough to fill the time when nothing else is more interesting?

3. Is your child's time delineated between what they want to do and what they need to do for someone else or even for them?

4. Are they multi-tasking?

Homework and self-directed projects get sabotaged when there is not enough choice and flexibility involved; when your child feels like what she is being asked to do has little or no personal value; when the task is given as a punishment or when the task involves high levels of thought-process repetitive tasks. Homework will often fit into this last category. For example, your child is learning how to add and subtract and she proves, at least to herself that she has the concept down after three or four problems, however, the homework has twenty problems. Therefore, with each problem your child completes after feeling masterful of the material (if she continues at all), she becomes more resentful and less attentive and finally just starts writing anything down. The first solution here is not to make all the math problems just straightforward numbers; word problems would be more challenging. Second is to break up the repetition by having your child do the problems in smaller chunks. Third, have your child complete a reasonable number of the problems and if she gets them all correct, allow her to be done. If all must be completed, finish them with her, engaging her as much as possible. Make it fun.

Set up all the homework and unfinished projects on a large (preferably round) table. As your child loses energy and interest in one, have your child do something to release any built up energies for two to three minutes (no more than five). Then, have your child walk around the table and choose the next thing on which she wants to work. When your child finishes something and it is done correctly and completely, either remove it or somehow indicate that your child has had a completion such as putting it up on the refrigerator, showing it to other people or discussing the work at dinner.

Supporting your child to get her homework done involves helping your child to create various structures, as well as taking note if there is a time pattern to how long your child can be successfully working on any one thing. Watch for fidgeting and a loss of focus; redirect your child back to the project or assignment or get your child to take one of her breaks. Make sure your child has recently taken an emotional coffee break before asking her to do tasks that are likely to create some frustration. Experiment with different times and different circumstances to see what seems to work best for your child. Keep track. Does your child do better when she gets some part or all of her homework done as soon as she gets home? Does she need a snack first or to release pent-up energy before beginning? Does she need some one on one refueling time with a trusted adult or older sibling or close friends before tackling the homework? Are there days that your child's patterns, once established, seem to get thrown for a loop? If so, what is different about those days? Does your child have gym or art or music those days? Are those days when an outside adult works with your child? When patterns emerge, or certain structuring habits seem more successful, keep track.

Guiding that child involves taking those observations and passing them on to your child to the extent your child is capable of handling them. Doing so begins to make your child more self-aware regarding what gives her good days and bad days and what works best and worst. Working within the action and consequences model makes your child more responsible for personal decisions once we know your child has the capability and necessary insights to make those decisions wisely. Guiding your child involves helping your child develop the critical thinking skills to do for herself.

Another way to support your child is to help her establish value between what she *needs* to do and what she *likes* to do. Help your child find value in learning the things that need to be learned when your child cannot see it for herself.

As parents really learn who their child is and how she functions in the world, they can then support her by being her interface with that world until she can do so independently. Guiding your child is teaching her how to advocate for herself and then standing first *with* her and then *behind* her as she does it on her own.

General Strategies

1. Identify the child's learning style.

2. Work with the child to find value and create interest.

3. Apply what you have learned by painting the portrait and knowing what engages the child.

4. Identify thought processing groups.

5. Rotate buddy style of learning.

6. Floating teacher facilitators. Let them teach to the whole class.

Physical Strategies

Steady Pattern

1. Simulate physical activity.

2. Allow movement breaks.

3. When the child finishes something, have the child come to you and give him directions on how to further his activities.

Pulse Pattern

1. Limit activities that simulate physical activity for more than 10 – 15 minutes at a time.

2. Allow frequent movement breaks.

3. When the child finishes something, have the child come to you and give him a physical activity to do.

4. Offer the child quiet, unobtrusive physical activity.

5. Sit the child in the back and end corners of the classroom

Crescendo Pattern

1. Gear activities to mirror the energy pattern.

2. Ask parents to help identify the child's rhythm.

General Physical Level Strategies

Teacher/Classroom

1. Eat less at a time but more frequently.

2. Take more breaks.

3. Work with the child's energy patterns.

4. Encourage drinking of water.

5. Have the child do "coded" errands.

6. Always have "busy work" ready.

7. Take music breaks.

8. Implement project corners.

9. Try various lighting scenarios.

10. Include the child in environmental concerns.

Teacher/Parent
1. Provide healthy foods & drinks for both school and home.

2. Eat less at a time but more frequently; emphasize the importance of breakfast.

3. Consider looking into an allergy/food sensitivity diet for the child.

Emotional Strategies

1. Pay attention to where and by whom the child is placed in the classroom.

2. Observe warning signs of impending drops.

3. Identify and address personality changes.

4. Provide the child with emotional coffee breaks.

Intellectual Strategies

Spaghetti

1. Ask questions that lead the child back to the subject at hand.

2. Verbally engage the child in conversation that brings him back; avoid one or two-word phrases.

3. Ask or help the child to find the value/interest in the topic at hand.

4. Vary your presentation style and fill it with surprises – keep the child guessing.

Pulse/Burst Strategies

1. Help the student create a "thought keeper" notebook.

2. Raise the challenge of the information.

3. Have the child connect their disconnected thoughts.

4. Teach the child to write in shorthand for thoughts or questions he has while you are teaching.

DSL

1. Have the child learn a color-coding system that matches like concepts and ideas.

2. Teach the child to create a shorthand which the child can utilize to quickly notate all the different things flowing through his awareness.

3. Teach the child "quieting the mind" exercises.

The following list of questions should always be in the forefront of creating educational plans for any child:

1. What are the child's natural gifts and talents?

2. Where do his interests lie?

3. How can you best connect a subject or an area where there is no interest to an area where there is an interest?

CHAPTER 6

TEACHING

Inventive Ways To Engage and Teach The ADD/HD Child

EVERYTHING OLD IS new again. We need to make learning for these children applicable to their lives and interactive in nature. Information needs to be taught in multiple learning formats that challenge and engage them. This can be done by engaging and developing their own critical thinking skills which gives them a feeling of ownership in the process.

If you are going to teach kids who live outside the box you need to teach them outside the box. Here are some ideas:

1. Teach them how to knit and crochet, at the youngest age possible, and through that venue teach them to count and learn about colors and shapes and patterns. By doing this, you are giving them something to do that they can work on while listening to other subjects. These are perfect activities that can start in day care or a preschool program as well as at home. It improves their physical dexterity and they create something in the process that they can show off or give away. It beats the hell out of squeezing a stress ball.

2. Teach them about fractions and wet and dry measurements through teaching them how to cook and measure. Also, while teaching them to cook, teach them about nutrition and food groups. Be sure the information is practical for them.

3. Have them learn history, geography, science, et cetera, through playing games on a Wii or something kinetic so they are getting physical activity while also learning.

4. Teach them science through teaching them how to garden. You can even cross over history, farming and games such as Farmville on Facebook.

5. Have them take turns co-teaching and tutoring.

6. Learn math through art and music as well as history.

7. By junior high school, have them setting up towns and villages to teach them about voting responsibly and democracy. Have them do elections; hold the elected accountable. Begin teaching them about career paths and choices. Engage small business owners to teach them entrepreneurship. Have them adopt a cause and raise money.

8. Create internships and or apprenticeships starting in junior high which interest the child and can be used to assign value in areas or subjects that the student struggles to find interest or value in.

9. Eliminate standardize testing. All testing should be conducted in a way that supports the students' different learning styles. All testing should be done orally, visually, and with interactive components.

10. Eliminate failing and staying back; recognize progress and effort. Always pair up the child in one of their areas of strength with someone who is struggling with that area so that they can teach/tutor them. Then in their areas of weakness find a good student match to assist them.

11. Create exercises where each student, on a regular basis, has to learn how to lead, how to follow, how to manage, how to delegate and how to be one of the primary workers.

12. Eliminate classrooms based on age; rather, base them on each child's level in each area with cross over so that those who are most excelled in any one area are helping others who struggle in the same area.

This is a partial list meant to stimulate the creative problem solving juices around new, better and different ways to engage all the gifts that these children have.

Next I would like to tackle one in particular that I feel does injustice to a great many children, ADD/HD or not, and that is number 9- Eliminate standardized testing. As I have always told my students, employees or anyone else who felt like I was responsible for the solution, don't bring me the problem without at least one solution in mind, give me a place to start and then we will problem solve it together. So here is the place to start on how to determine whether children are actually learning what we are trying to teach them.

Proof of Proficiency Learning

As we have become increasingly attached to the concept that testing is some panacea which guarantees that we have done our job in education we continually avoid a simple and sometimes painful truth that passing a test is not as much the demonstration of learning about something in a utilizable way as much as it is the ability to memorize. I have often referred to the current education system as the vomit system of learning, as long as the child takes the information in and vomits it out in the right order they get a pat on the head and a kick in the backsides and is moved forward. However, has the child actually interacted with the information, do that have a working application of the knowledge, can they do something with it, out of the context of the memorization of it?

Standardized testing has created more problems than it has solved and it certainly has not indicated that the student that can pass one is truly ready for college, or is prepared to be out in the world or even ready for the next grade. Standardized testing does not indicate either intelligence or the lack of it, however it does measure the ability to memorize. All of the emphasis on memorization based learning only develops certain areas of the brain. The brain, like a muscle, develops best through exercises that involve *cross training* of brain functions just like the body develops better and is overall more fit and able by working all its muscle groups. In muscle group terms children today may have one hell of a right bicep and some upper body strength but have no leg muscle on which to take those things that they are learning anywhere.

These are my recommendations for a more accurate way to determine whether children are really developing skill sets, acquiring knowledge, and learning how to think rather than passing or failing at memorizing information and replicating processes with no true understanding or skill set development.

1. We need to develop assessments of understanding that is equally divided up in testing that is done orally, written and through demonstration.

2. We need to have that assessment of understanding include cross usage of the topic or subject.

3. They need to teach the information to someone else, which will show a deeper level of understanding and comprehension of the subject.

4. They need to take the information and shows ways it applies in their world or the greater world at large.

5. Have them analytically explain abstract concepts have them abstractly demonstrate (physical, expressive or creative) analytical concepts creating stronger links between the left and right brain.

6. Do something in a group or team setting with the information.

Eliminate the current grading system and replace it with the following assessment system of the child's progress:

Innovator Ability	IA	They have the ability to take what they learn and shift or change it in a way that is beyond what they have been taught.
Teacher Ability	TA	This is an indication of a level of mastery of the information which means they could teach it in all three learning formats.
Exceeds Expectation	EE	This indicates they are ahead of the overall class and could teach it in one to two areas.
Demonstrates Understanding	DU	They can perform the actions or give the explanation that shows they understand the concept but do not have the ability to teach it. However, they do have some capacity to cross apply and shift it around. This shows that the child can demonstrate some critical thinking skills in this area.
Working Knowledge	WK	They show have the knowledge and can work with it in the most basic of ways.
Work in Progress	WP	They need some additional support which needs to be done both at home and at school.
New Approach Needed	NAN	This child needs a different approach and/or teacher to help them with this concept.

This kind of assessment system gives us more information that helps the educator and parent to see where strengths, weakness, talents, gifts and shortcomings are. Looking at these closer, we are not creating a child-centered pass or fail mentality. We also, as time goes on, have more information with which teachers and parents can guide the child to not only areas they have interest, but how to use their strengths within that area.

In this system we go one step further and also establish whether the child falls into one of the following categories: Doer, Teacher, Facilitator or Innovator. These categories fall on a spectrum; they will shift from subject to subject and are also indicators of what fields or areas of expertise the child is headed for. It also may help choose certain proficiencies or jobs within an area. These are the natural roles that your child will play depending on the subject and the buy in. If there is no buy in and no value, worth or engagement created within the child then they are either apathetic, frustrated or angry, depending on how much they are being pushed and how much of their value has been assigned to the successful completion of the task.

The level of connectedness that they feel to the project, task or information and how much they attached to it will determine whether they are passive or active in their role.

Doer

The passive doer is a *follower,* who will function well with specific, consistent, persistent guidance. For the active doer, you just wind them up and let them go. If they are also high in energies of teacher or facilitator, then they may step up to the role of working manger or group leader. I call these the *accidental leaders,* who because of their energy and enthusiasm people just follow them whether they want to be followed or not.

Teacher

Teachers, on the passive end of the spectrum, can articulate the information when asked in at least one or more formats and are willing to do it, but do not necessarily seek it out. Whereas active Teachers enjoys teaching and showing, and can naturally make adjustments if the person who they are trying to teach is struggling with the learning to the ultimate Teacher on the opposite end of the spectrum who can't help themselves, are always teaching, explaining, and showing and helping everyone around them.

Facilitator

Facilitators want to make things work. From the passive end of the spectrum where they simply want things to work in and for their world, to the active end, where they want to make things work for everyone in their world all the way to the extreme end where they just want to make things work period, everywhere, everything, period. Depending on their social skills, they are your managers by consensus, and group leaders, not ring leaders, but group leaders. Facilitators will have more of a tendency to change the system by shifting, stretching and changing it then rebelling against it. They are diplomats and politicians.

Innovator

Innovators are driven by the energies to either invent and create or re-invent and re-re-create. If passive, they can be isolated loners who are far more interested in the possibilities within than realities as they are being presented. In their active state they are innovating through interaction which may show up with strong teaching energies or facilitating energies and all the way to leading the charge. Innovators are leaders who many times can also be known as rebels, troublemakers or even heretics.

A child may be a low level Doer, at best, in one area, yet an Innovator or Teacher extraordinaire in another. Obviously the latter area is the one where you may glimpse the child's career or vocation in life. The ability to infuse, through showing the interconnectedness of knowledge and where the things they struggle with can apply or help with the things they are passionate about, is the cornerstone of the child's individual educational plan. Don't confuse what I just said with the school's version of an IEP (Individual Educational plan) but the is the Individual educational and life plan that the parent should be weaving for the child, to help them succeed.

I have worked on IEP plans with schools and my clients. They often talk more about what is going to be achieved by the student and less on how it is going to actually happen. The suggestions are within very defined boundaries that often, until they medicate, seem to have little effect on any significant, consistent changes or improvements. Ergo medicate. But what if the lack of improvement does not indicate medication as much as a better recommenda-tion, deeper understanding of what the child needs and a way of learning and being in the world. It is not uncommon to hear how these medicated individuals loose parts of themselves while being medicated. Sure they can focus better but are not achieving their fullest potential, what they achieve is separating themselves from enough if their brilliance and creativity to stay focused on the mediocrity of what they are learning. They are more patient with the slowness of the pace or the inaneness of the information. Which tells us that something is being lost, held back or separated out which is part of these children's gifts.

The sad part is some of the things that they can't focus on because it registers as inane, boring or uninteresting are things that might be none of those things if it was presented in ways that engaged them more. We medicate more and more because of a broken system of education than because that it is the only or the best option for these children.

Some Additional Thoughts

As I have traveled around talking about some of the things I would change or do with the education system which would help these children learn, thrive and grow, without medication or loss of self, self-worth and self-esteem, I have been told that these methods and ways of educating would help any child. However, that was usually followed by the list of reasons why creating this kind of education system for our children would be impossible. To that I respond, if we keep trying to fix something that is beyond repair over the long run not only we will spend more money and time and use up more resources to never get significantly better results but also sooner or later we will have to make the change. We must set the bar where it belongs - high. It is the future of our children, our country, humanity itself, we are talking about. Can we really afford to not make the change? Can we continue to support a system where as long as those in power finically benefit that we will turn a blind eye? Can we look our children in the faces in 20 or 30 years with a clear conscience when the larger effects of drug'em up and dumb'em down mentality begin to haunt them and us? When the physical, emotional and societal effects become undeniable, will we look to these children and honestly be able to say that we did our best?

CHAPTER 7

TAKING A CLOSER LOOK AT THE DIAGNOSTIC AND STATISTICAL MANUAL (DSM-IV)

S O WHAT ARE we talking about here when we use the term ADHD? Well, below is the description out of the Diagnostic and Statistical Manual IV, with a few comments from me along the way...as always.

Numeric codes indicating type based on criteria (adapted from *DSM-IV-TR*) are as follows:

- *314.00 ADHD: Predominantly inattentive type if inattention criterion is met for the past 6 months, but hyperactivity/impulsivity criterion is not met*

If the hyperactivity/impulsivity criterion is not met then why is it called Attention Deficit Hyperactivity Disorder? I wonder if it is because it has become unfashionable to medicate kids with just ADD?

- *314.01 ADHD: Predominantly hyperactive/impulsive type if hyperactivity/impulsivity criterion is met for the past 6 months, but inattention criterion is not met.*

If the inattention criteria not met why is it called Attention Deficit Hyperactivity Disorder?

- *314.01 ADHD: Combined type if both inattention and hyperactivity/impulsivity criteria are met for past 6 months (Note that this code is the same as that used for the predominantly hyperactive type.)*

How important is the issue of the inattention if the code is the same whether it exists or not? Is there more of a push for medication because of hyperactivity then for inattention? Does someone monitor which codes should be medicated and which shouldn't be?

- *314.9 ADHD not otherwise specified (NOS): Other disorders with prominent symptoms of attention-deficit or hyperactivity-impulsivity that do not meet DSM-IV-TR criteria.*

This leaves the door open so the criteria don't have to be met yet the label can be applied and of course medicated.

The determination of whether these codes are applicable or not are fully dependent upon observation. Observations are made mostly by people who are emotionally attached to either the individual, or have a vested interest in the situation that the individual is involved in, less so in the case of an adult but most certainly in the case of a child. From a parental stand point that can skew the observations from either prospective. Is it reasonable to expect a parent to be unbiased? A parent might play down certain behaviors but it is far more likely, especially depending upon the demographic of the household, that certain traits associated with ADD/HD are exacerbated, perhaps to the point where a diagnosis is needed because it appears as if medication is the only option. Households with higher percentage rates of children being diagnosed and medicated are single parent, poorer, less educated households. Households were children are more likely to eat less healthy and have less quality adult interaction. These are also households who are more likely to get subsidies or help in paying for the medication. Less educated, financially struggling, and stressed out single parents are really good impartial observers or advocates for their child's needs.

Let's look at the other group of observers whom are making these determinations, educators. Don't educators have a vested interest in a better managed, quieter classroom? They know that a medicated child is a child who will not be jumping around, jumping ahead and asking out of sequence questions, or questioning answers. Educators, who are being under -funded and pressured to produce results through a questionable model (standardized test scores) with overcrowded classrooms and oftentimes little or no support from over-stressed, over-worked parents, are the other observers.

Genetics

- *Parents and siblings of children with ADHD are 2-8 times more likely to develop ADHD than the general population, suggesting that ADHD is a highly familial disease.*

For over a decade, I have been saying that this thing we are calling ADD/HD is part of an evolutionary process, that it started coming in the mid 1800s and that the early ADD/HD individuals were the architects of the 21st century.

In their day, many of these individuals didn't do well in the education system or fit in well with society. They were often considered the village idiot at best and trouble makers at worst. Because institutions such as public education, pharmaceutical lobbyists, the American Medical Association & American Psychological Association did not have the stranglehold they have now through their placement within and access to government, these individuals were left to go their own way.

Along the way, they gave us telegraphs, telephones, radios, computers automobiles, and more technology, artistry, philosophy, and insights then I could list here — all without medication.

Inattention

Must include at least 6 of the following symptoms of inattention that must have persisted for at least 6 months to a degree that is maladaptive and inconsistent with developmental level:

- *Often fails to give close attention to details or makes careless mistakes in schoolwork, work, or other activities.*

Bored, disinterested, has not been shown a value in the task that are being asked of them.

- *Often has difficulty sustaining attention in tasks or play activities.*

Lost interest or see above.

- *Often does not seem to listen to what is being said.*

What is going on in their head is more interesting than what is being said to them or they are being talked at instead of being engaged and talked with.

- *Often does not follow through on instructions and fails to finish schoolwork, chores, or duties in the workplace (not due to oppositional behavior or failure to understand instructions).*

Bored, disinterested, has not been shown a value in the task that are being asked of them, were not part of the creation process.

- *Often has difficulties organizing tasks and activities*

This mind needs just enough structure to fly, not enough and it can't get off the ground, too much and it feels strangled and will destruct the structure. Organizational tools need to be set-up interactively, engaging the individual to the value of them.

- *Often avoids or strongly dislikes tasks (such as schoolwork or homework) that require sustained mental effort.*

Bored, disinterested or unengaged. A critical thinking based, interactive, multiple learning style, multiple intelligence based approach would be far more successful than the "sit, beg & roll over" format we currently use.

- *Often loses things necessary for tasks or activities (school assignments, pencils, books, tools, or toys).*

Tools need to be put in place to manage the amount of stimuli that these individuals are processing on a number of different levels. Also, diet and environment can be a factor here.

- *Often is easily distracted by extraneous stimuli.*

What is going on in their head is more interesting than what is being said to them or they are being talked at instead of being engaged and talked with. Also, a bad diet and environmental factors can cause this.

- *Often forgetful in daily activities*

There are two settings for the ADD/HD child, hyper-focus and multi-task. Hyper-focus is when you have caught their attention and interest, they have been challenged in some way and will follow through to an internal level of satisfaction those things they are hyper-focused on. When they have reached a point where it is no longer interesting or that they can see where the "trip of learning about" is taking them, it is time for them to move on to something else.

As you were reading the above information, you will note that I put some thoughts by each criteria. Many of these approaches, however would take a much more time and resource intensive way of parenting, teaching and supporting these individuals. The question is: will the pay off of getting the additional insight, brilliance and creativity, to name a few, that we get through this extra set of efforts outweigh the extra effort it takes to educate them, or should we just continue to force medicate them because it is easier on us?

Hyperactivity/Impulsivity

Must include at least 4 of the following symptoms of hyperactivity-impulsivity that must have persisted for at least 6 months to a degree that is maladaptive and inconsistent with developmental level:

- *Hyperactivity evidenced by fidgeting with hands or feet, squirming in seat.*

Diet, environment, and lack of opportunity to deal with energy.

- *Hyperactivity evidenced by leaving seat in classroom or in other situations in which remaining seated is expected.*

See above, it is a fair expectation?

- *Hyperactivity evidenced by running about or climbing excessively in situations where this behavior is inappropriate (in adolescents or adults, this may be limited to subjective feelings of restlessness).*

Diet, environment, and lack of opportunity to deal with energy. Also, more coping tools need to be put in place to deal with the increase of stimuli these children experience on all levels.

- *Hyperactivity evidenced by difficulty playing or engaging in leisure activities quietly.*

Is there enough engagement of the mind as well as enough physical releases? We also need to look at diet and reactions to toxic environmental factors.

- *Impulsivity evidenced by blurting out answers to questions before the questions have been completed.*

Bored – the pace of the information is not fast enough to keep them engaged and excited because they are often are seen as not bright. Also, check diet and environment.

- *Impulsivity evidenced by showing difficulty waiting in lines or awaiting turn in games or group situations.*

Lack of planning, too high an expectation for the level of the individual, tools needed, diet and environment.

I have put a heavy emphasis on diet and environment in this section, but I am talking about both what they are and are not getting enough of in their diet. Environmental factors can be anything from the physical (lightening, smells, chemicals) to the emotional and the mental. If we could look more often at hyperactivity as an allergic reaction, in a broader sense of the word and began to address the triggers of that reaction, then maybe medication would not be necessary at all.

General Criteria

- *Onset is no later than age 7 years.*

By recognizing ADD/AD as an evolutionary process, this is a no brainer. However, visual learners can often fall through the net depending on what the impacts are on the emotional, physical and energetic levels.

- *Symptoms must be present in 2 or more situations, such as school, work, or home.*

How many different situations are there for symptoms to show up before the age of seven, and if there are that many situations, then is ADD/HD the issue? Also in my experience, the child can be seen as challenging but manageable at home, but it is the educational system's pressure that pushes for the label and medication. So if these children are manageable at home but not at school, then is ADD/HD really the issue we should be looking at?

- *The disturbance causes clinically significant distress or impairment in social, academic, or occupational functioning.*

In "Managing the Gift: Alternative Approaches For Attention Deficit Disorder" I spoke of how instead of naming it ADD, we should have called it C.I.S.- Cultural Inconvenience Syndrome, for as often as not that is truly why we are medicating them.

- *Disorder does not occur exclusively during the course of a pervasive developmental disorder, schizophrenia, or other psychotic disorder and is not better accounted for by mood, anxiety, dissociative, or personality disorder.*

If only the threads were all that simple. Self-worth, self-esteem, shame, anxiety, fear, depression and isolation are all side effects as bi-products of an ADD individual living in a non-ADD world.

How much of what our kids are experiencing is because of our handling of a situation within them that we do not fully understand or as Heinlein would say "GROK". We just don't grok them so we punish them for not fitting into social and academic situations which are as foreign to them as the earth was to Michael Valentine Smith, the human Martian in "Stranger in a Strange Land." Even though he had an innocence and apparent lack of social skills or understanding when he first landed, does this mean he wasn't as bright, or as good or as able as those around him, or was he simply a stranger in a strange land? In the end, he was quite a bit smarter and wiser then his human counterparts because he saw the world differently, from a different set of eyes, a different perspective. So do many of these kids, but they don't know how to verbalize it, sometimes within themselves or to others. Things that we accept without questioning, do not make sense to them, and they challenge us with their very different way of seeing and being. We have never in all of recorded history treated differences very well, we persecute and punish people, cultures and belief systems that we do not understand, and are not our own.

Perhaps we are more culturally advanced, urban and better at manipulating truths then we used to be. However, I fear that our predecessors will still find our treatment of ADD/HD individuals, in the later part of the 20th century and beginning of the 21st century, to be acts of little tolerance for differences. Also, they will view our cashing in on these children as aberrant behavior and an indicator as a psychologically ill society where greed and power were still more important than the care and support of our children or the future of our planet or humanity itself. But unlike the animals that we drive into extinction through our acts of greed or the eco-systems we destroy, these kids will live to fight back against the way they were treated.

Mental Status Examination may note the following:

- *Appearance: Most often, appointments are difficult to structure and maintain due to hyperactivity and distractibility. Children with ADHD may present as fidgety, impulsive, and unable to sit still, or they may actively run around the office. Adults with ADHD may be distractible, fidgety, and forgetful.*

It takes time to find the right amount of structure for these children to be productive and even receptive in. Also, until one has numerous interactions, understands the outside factors which may be affecting the child's performance, whether in the classroom, the home or the a professional's office it is easy to jump to conclusions. In addition, I suspect there is not enough weight given to the increasing anxiety that exists within the child who is more and more singled out, reprimanded and repeatedly "observed". Fitting in as part of the family and social unit, what I like to call "the tribe" is of utmost importance especially when the child is given messages that indicate to them that their place may be in danger within that tribe.

- *Affect/mood: Affect usually is appropriate and may be elevated, but it should not be euphoric. Mood usually is euthymic, except for periods of low self-esteem and decreased (dysthymic) mood. Mood and affect are not primarily affected by ADHD, although irritability may frequently be associated with ADHD.*

If the people who are there to teach you and help you discover who you are, what your gifts are and where your place in the world is, are not only unable to help you do so but are punishing you for their failure to help, wouldn't you be irritable too?

- *Speech/thought processes: Speech is of normal rate but may be louder due to impulsivity. Thought processes are goal-directed but may reflect difficulties staying on a topic or task. Evidence of racing thoughts or pressured speech should not be present. These symptoms are more consistent with a manic state (bipolar disorder).*

Heightened sensitivity to the energies around them can cause louder and more distracted speech.

- *Hallucinations or delusions: Not present.*

- *Thought content/suicide: Content should be normal, with no evidence of suicidal/homicidal or psychotic symptoms.*

- *Cognition: Concentration and storage into recent memory are affected. Patients with ADHD may have difficulty with calculation tasks and recent memory tasks. Orientation, remote memory, or abstraction should not be affected.*

ADHD is associated with a number of other clinical diagnoses. Studies have demonstrated that many individuals have both ADHD and antisocial personality disorder (ASD).[10] These individuals are at higher risk for self-injurious behaviors. ADHD is also linked to addictive behavior. The more severe the symptoms of ADHD, the greater the use of tobacco, alcohol, and marijuana.[11]- Some individuals have both ADHD and an autism spectrum disorder.[12]

I would caution parents who start lining up multiple diagnoses not to move into medication-based solutions. It has become a more common practice to create and adjust "drug cocktails" until they get the desired behavior, which may or may not have anything to do with what is in the best interest of the child and can have severe long term side effects.

Find a health care advocate for your team who looks at all sides of the problems and is in alignment with your desire to have what is in the best interest of the child, not the best interest of those serving the child and to keep it as healthy and natural as possible.

Symptoms of ADHD and bipolar disorder may be directly correlated. Patients with ADHD should be assessed for possible underlying or coexisting bipolar disorder, and vice versa.

Environment

- *Hypotheses exist that include in utero exposures to toxic substances, food additives or colorings, or allergic causes. However, diet, especially sugar, is not a cause of ADHD.*

Here is a place where again we need to look at the difference between the impacts/gifts of ADD/HD and the environmental exacerbation of those impacts/gifts. Why would we think that exposure to *"toxic substances, food additives or colorings, or allergic causes"* can create negative effects on any baby in utero but we need to separate those effects from what is purely ADD/HD.

As far as sugar goes there is a plethora of information about the dangers of the overuse of sugar in everyone's diet and the issues of the negative impacts of the sugar addiction cycle. Looking at the things that are associated with that high lower roller coaster ride of the drug sugar, it could certainly create those negative behaviors associated with ADD/HD. So if you then take behaviors that are manageable without medication and add the sugar cycle and they become unmanageable, is it an ADD/HD issue?

How much of a role family environment has in the pathogenesis of ADHD is unclear, but it certainly may exacerbate symptoms.

What goes on at home MAY exacerbate how the child acts out in school or out of the home- sorry that is simply too stupid to even justify a response, except for maybe, Duh!

CHAPTER 8

MEDICATIONS, MANIPULATION, MONEY AND MUSINGS

I N THIS CHAPTER, I have included statistical data I found interesting, and comments, articles and blog posts from myself and about the ADD/HD issue that is facing America today. I hope you find these interesting and informative. Why am I sharing other people's blogs and articles? Because I know what I do well and what I don't. Research is not my thing. I am a hands-on person, who through the blending of intuitive and intellect has helped people with ADD/HD to better understand it. Also, I do not like reinventing the wheel so when I do find things and blog about them, why restructure it. So here they are.

Managing the Gift

As ADD/HD medications have become multi-million dollar a year industry, more of what we are told and what information is shared with us and how it is shared definitely has been increasingly influenced by whether or not it positively affects the ADD/HD cash flow game.

One of my earlier blogs addressed just this. Back in 2000-2001, I, the Merrow Report (PBS), and a few other isolated voices were trying to sound the alarms about the questionable reliability of information out of such places as

CHADD (the largest non-profit organization for the support of ADD/HD) or millions of dollars spent on a government program that got yanked at the last moment whose messages always came back to the "don't forget the medication" message when the major backers, funders and/or donors were the drug companies that profited off of the sale of ADD/HD drugs.

I was talking on any show that would have me or any event where I could speak about what I felt were horrifying statistics. Between 1995-2000 there was a 400% increase of prescriptions written for ADD/HD drugs for 2-4 year olds, when the Physician's Desk Reference said that it was not recommended for any child under the age of eight. The number of ADD/HD medication related deaths had by that time eclipsed the number of deaths caused by the misuse of the herb Ephedra, which had been pulled off the market for being too dangerous, so why the double standard? School systems at the time were blackmailing parents into medicating their kids (until stricter laws came into place). But the numbers of kids (and later adults) were just not high enough to force changes, even if the issue was on the front covers of *Time* and *Newsweek*.

Being patriotic, terrorism and whether the state got to define whose God was allowed to make the rules as to what we called marriage, were the issues, not whether we were over-medicating our children to hide deeper, more troubling problems like the sad state of public education, the family unit and a government whose dedication to its top lobbyist cash flow were more important than its dedication to our children. Now, 10 years later, we have had unusual double-digit growth in diagnosis of ADD/HD and some years, even triple digit growth in the numbers of kids being medicated for it.

What I want to do over the next several blogs is to locate some of the current information out there, share it with you, comment on it, and sometimes even give you a different perspective. I am not saying that medication should never be used, I have always said it should be the absolute last choice and only used after all other things, that don't have side effects, have been put into place. But we should not make it the first choice, or just an easy way out.

Is medication successful? It depends on your definition. If you want to define success as by the drugging of these kids, it makes it easier to sustain a broken education system, then the answer is an unequivocal yes. If we define success as helping these children to become more self-aware of their choices, reaching more or their potentials, supporting them to higher and greater levels of thought, creativity and utilize their gifts in the fullest of ways, then the answer is no. Fast food answers and quick fixes don't solve problems, they just make them easier to avoid.

Everybody is Making Money on ADHD, But at What Cost?

I just finished reading a disturbing, but not surprising article by John Grohol (http://psychcentral.com/blog/archives/2010/12/13/ssi-encourages-families-to-label-healthy-children-with-adhd-as-disabled/) about how parents are being encouraged to get their children labeled as being disabled, and therefore medicated, in order to collect SSI benefits. Thirty one percent of those receiving benefits have children labeled with ADHD, the number one disorder.

We now have a system where everyone gets to make money on ADHD, which of course is paid for by a government that is bankrupt. So let's follow this through a little, shall we?

For a child to be labeled as ADHD is not enough. In order for the family to get funds and services, the federal government mandates that they HAVE to be medicated in order to qualify. In his article, Grohol pointed out: *"One of the most disturbing parts of the program seems to be the mandate by federal government officials who administer the program that in order for a child to be considered seriously disabled (at least in the government's eyes), they need to be on psychiatric medications — whether the parents wants them to be or not"*

The parents receive on average more benefits (sometimes twice as much) than if they were just on welfare.

Everyone involved in the labeling process is making money, paid in most cases by the system — in other words, the taxpayer.

The doctor who writes the prescription and the pharmaceutical companies get their built in regular paycheck guaranteed.

The school system gets additional funding for each disabled child they serve in their district, whether they are providing the needed services or not. Yes, they follow the letter of the law and provide the paperwork and meetings required for qualification. But the number of kids that are actually receiving beneficial help is a much murkier question.

A medicated child (drug 'em up and dumb 'em down) needs less help and attention in the classroom, helping to support the idea of schools having larger classrooms.

So, the education system remains broken. It receives increased funding through increasing the number of disabled children in their system. The drug companies get to profit off these diagnoses, as well as several other providers, most of who are providing only band-aids of service and usually have regular ongoing profits with no exit strategy involved. Then we have a family struggling with how to not lose their house and how to afford food and being told that they can now qualify for free money from the government if they will simply drug their child.

On the surface, this approach makes everyone's life easier and helps a whole lot of money stay in flow in the economy.

But why does our government refuse to support non-medicated based solutions to an issue that for many is still in question as a true diagnosis at all? Simple, in 2010 the pharmaceutical/health product industry was the single largest contributing lobbyist group, who by the third quarter of last year had spent over 186 million dollars to make sure that their issues and protections and tax benefits were staying in place. This is 45 million more than the next group (electric utilities) and almost 2.5 times more than the education lobby. I did notice that there was no lobby group for children or under funded families. Oh well, it's only a couple hundred thousand kids are being sacrificed, and if it keeps Washington well oiled and pharmaceutical company share holder profits high, what the hell!

Why All the Focus on Medications?

When you hear about ADD/ADHD, you usually hear about medication sooner or later... usually sooner. Most of the time, the person sings the praises of medication. However, an increasing set of voices is less thrilled with the medication options.

Parents want to know about long term health effects of medications. They wonder, "Exactly what do these ADD medications do?" Many people ask why some of these medications are similar to speed. That seems like giving a child a line of coke to snort. How can that be healthy?

Other people wonder if behavior modification drugs increase the risk of children self-medicating when they become teen-agers? In addition, do other problems get lost in the medicating?

Are these concerns valid? Here are some things I have discovered in my research:

Between the years of 1990 and 2000, over 569 children were hospitalized in ADD/ADHD medication-related incidents, 38 of them were life threatening hospitalizations, and 186 died. Some people claim that number is now over a thousand.

The FDA has issued reports on the top three ADD/ADHD drugs, Adderall, Concerta and Ritalin.

Adderall (extended release) was linked to 20 sudden deaths, 14 of whom were children. Adderal Extended Release was withdrawn from market by Health Canada.

Concerta (methylphenidate, similar to Ritalin) is linked to difficulty breathing, irregular, fast heartbeat, high blood pressure, and liver damage.

Related ADHD medications may also raise questions. For example, Strattera (atomoxetine) is linked to high systolic blood pressure, tachycardia, hypotension, abdominal pain, nausea, vomiting and mood swings. Even the Strattera website reports, "In some children and teens, Strattera increases the risk of suicidal thoughts."

After testing Concerta and Adderall, Dr. William Pelham noted results from a trial comparing drug and behavioral, non-drug approaches to ADHD. He found that 75% of children functioned well without ADHD drugs for a full year, as well as the year following the study. According to Dr. Pelham, "What this means to me is that two-thirds of ADHD kids could be taken off the medications."

Do those figures alarm you? They prompted me to continue my research into the use and risks of ADD/ADHD medications.

Since 1990, the number of people taking Ritalin has increased by 500%. As of early 2008, the United States has the highest level of Ritalin use and production.

Canada's Ritalin figures are under half of what the U.S. uses. No other countries have come close.

7 - 10% of American boys are on this drug, which is an overwhelming number compared to other countries around the world. The financial side of

this is especially disturbing. As a result of profits from the sale of Ritalin, the U.S. government makes over $450 million annually.

In over ten years of working with ADD/ADHD individuals, I have noticed that the evidence against ADD/ADHD medications has become more and more alarming. However, the numbers of kids diagnosed and medicated just continues to increase.

During that same time, we've seen pharmaceutical profits increase by double- and triple-digits. It's no surprise that pharmaceutical companies have increased their budgets for state and national lobbyists. Is this to keep ADHD-related medications off the table for FDA review?

In my experience, the attractiveness (just one pill) and cost (insurance covered) continue to make medication a popular choice.

Tell parents that they'll need to work with a different diet and attitudes. They'll need to develop new and time-intensive ways of parenting. Say that parents may have to fight a school system that often relies on medications as a solution, and the parents' responsibilities can seem a bit too much.

Then tell parents that their child will also have to learn new skill sets to deal with the world. Suddenly, one simple pill seems like a faster, easier solution. In addition, institutions such as educational, medical and social services reward the "correct" choice of medication.

What about the consequences? America seems to have lost some of its own skill sets. Harder work now can result in greater, longer term rewards through harder work now, but many parents choose the short-term fix instead. Our society has become accustomed to immediate gratification, and simple solutions with the ease of a drive-thru window.

If all else fails, there's blame. We've become very good at it. If our child becomes a drug addict – or worse -- so what? We can blame the doctors, the educators who supported the medications, and the pharmaceutical companies. If we are real lucky we can even find someone to sue. That's the American way... isn't it?

If you're shuddering at that idea, there are answers. Successful non-drug treatments exist, and – as Dr. Pelham's studies suggest – they can work as well or better than ADD/ADHD medications. Throughout the traditional and alternative health care fields, an increasing number of experts offer non-drug solutions and coaching. Between community resources and online referrals, you can find help.

Don't wait for a health crisis with your child. The healthiest solutions aren't as easy as a single pill, but the long-term benefits of alternative approaches are more than worthwhile.

For Whose Benefit Do We Drug Our Children?

Has Ritalin entered the Guinness Book of World Records?

Is there a contest for prescription drug use among children?

According to the Boston Globe newspaper, "New Englanders buy more of the stimulant Ritalin and its generic equivalents per capita than residents of any other part of the country, a fact that prescribers attribute to the region's affluence and access to medical care."

When I read that, I feel stuck between sadness and outrage.

Sound like a good thing that we give our children more of a drug, that is a stimulant (speed) than anywhere else in the country. It is so nice to know that we are so medically advanced that we can drug our kids into fitting into an archaic 19th century school model. Where the majority of learning is still based on what I call- "the intellectual version of vomiting." That is, memorize what you're taught. Learn it in the correct order, spit it up in the right order, get a pat on the head and then move on.

Of the ten top states, the Globe goes on to report; New Hampshire is number one in the country, followed by Vermont, Massachusetts, Rhode Island and Maine. All in the top ten. Good medical care or a convenient way to not have to provide the services that a non-medicated child would require, in order to live up to the mandatory testing that the school systems have to pass, to continue to get funding?

Did the author at the Boston Globe look at the side effects? How about the lawsuits? Has she talked to any of the parents of children who are or were "emotionally blackmailed" or "veiled threatened" into medicating their child? How about that between 1990-1997 that there were 160 deaths associated with the use of Ritalin? And that was before the numbers of children taking got to the levels they are now.

That national magazines, law makers, even some members of the educational system, medical doctors and the psychiatric community are questioning whether ADD/ADHD is the epidemic or the giving out of medication. The production of Ritalin has increased 700% since 1990. The number of children on the medication is, estimated by some, to be reaching the 4 million mark. Others have put it as high as 5 million and as there are an estimated 8 million children, school aged, who are on psychiatric drugs (Breeding, 2000). Of course that doesn't count the two to five years olds who are now being put on Ritalin.

How can teaching children that the schools (and their life) should be a drug free zone when they are lining up in the halls ways to get their mid-morning dose of speed?

And what is Ritalin? We are told often that it is a mild stimulant of the central nervous system. Here is a more accurate definition, in the words of a 1995 drug enforcement agency (DEA) background paper on Ritalin- known as Methylphenidate. "Methylphenidate is a central nervous system (CNS) stimulant and shares many of the pharmacological effects of amphetamine, metamphetamine, and cocaine." It went on to state that Methylphenidate "produces behavioral, psychological, subjective, and reinforcing effects similar to those of d-amphetamine including increases in rating of euphoria, drug liking and activity, and decreases in sedation."

In 1995 the *Archives of General Psychiatry*, "Cocaine, which is one of the most reinforcing and addicting of the abused drugs, has pharmacological actions that are very similar to those of methylphenidate, which is now the most commonly prescribed psychotropic medicine for children in the U.S."

In *Driven to Distraction, it states that* "people with ADD feel focused when they take cocaine, just as they do when they take Ritalin."

We are often led to believe that Ritalin is non-addictive. The evidence is not supporting that idea. According to the book *Ritalin Nation:* "In 1994, Ritalin was the fastest growing amphetamine being used "non-medically" by high school seniors in Texas." Also that "children between 10 and 14 years old were involved in only about 25 emergency room visits connected with Ritalin abuse. In 1995, just four years later, that number had climbed to more than 400 visits, which for this group is about the same number of visits as for cocaine" And it also points out that "from 1990 to 1995, the DEA reports, there were about 2,000 thefts of methylphenidate, most of them night break-ins at pharmacies" - meaning that the drug "ranks in the top 10 most frequently reported pharmaceutical drugs diverted from licensed handlers." And at a special hearing of the Texas State Board of Education Gretchen Fuessner, a DEA pharmacologist, who assured the Board that it was a substance controlled and monitored by her agency exactly because of its proven addictive potential. Fuessner also presented data showing that up to 20% of young people with psychiatric prescription abuse their prescribed drug.

Don't get me wrong, medicine can be a good choice, when it is the last choice and everything else has been tried. But that is not the order of things. Let's put the child on speed- with indiscernible long-term side effects. Side effects? Long Term? Well the long-term results are too early to assess. And why would there be any long-term side effects with taking a small, developing and still growing body and putting speed into it on a daily basis. No, there won't be any side effects?

Besides so many things can hide behind daily doses of speed- traumas at home, at school, health issues, allergies and so much more. All easily swept away in a mind-numbing, robot like haze through medication.

What about the 2-4 year olds, whose prescriptions for Ritalin have sky-rocketed? The Physician's Desk Reference (PDR) says that Ritalin is not recommended for children under the age of six. Are those some of the stunning figures that allows us as a region (New England) or as a state (New Hampshire)? We medicate two year olds for being too active, aren't they suppose to be? Did the roles change? Are we abdicating our roles as parents, educators and members of the medical community to a pill bottle because it makes it easier? Easier for whom? And at what cost?

Parents may want to ask themselves to whom is their responsibility- their child or keeping the school system happy? Supporting overcrowded classrooms and antiquated learning methods by allowing them to medicate their child for the ease of the classroom.

FDA Approved Drugs[6]

Ritalin is the most and first prescribed drug for ADD/HD. The generic name is Methylphenidate. Ritalin has been used the longest, and has been

---

6 http://bigbassboca.blogspot.com/2011/01/first-blog-of-new-year.html
Note: Donna Bass has her degree in Behavioral Neuroscience and Psychobiology. She is currently working towards her Ph.D in Psychology.

found to be the most effective medication for ADD/HD, so the most information is available about it. Concerta is methylphenidate in an osmotic pump for metered dosage. Daytrana is also methylphenidate in patch form. However, in our quest for the quick fix, researchers are now finding that this fix does not come without a cost. The cost is our children's long term mental health. We as parents MUST be advocates for our children and in that vein, we need to be as educated as possible.

Carlezon and Anderson [1] have found that rats that were exposed to methylphenidate at a young age were in later life less able to experience pleasure and reward, and were more prone to despair / stress behaviors as adults.

In 2009, a call from NIDA to study Methylphenidate more comprehensively went something like this: "Methylphenidate, which is thought to be a fairly innocuous compound, can have structural and biochemical effects in some regions of the brain that can be even greater than those of cocaine," stated Dr.Yong Kim, lead author of the study. "Further studies are needed to determine the behavioral implications of these changes and to understand the mechanisms by which these drugs affect synapse formation" [2]

What does that mean in English? I'm not going to go ALL technical on you, but there is something here that needs to be made very, very clear. The brain of children, adolescents, and adults are very different from each other. This website has a very nice overview of the development of the brain: http://faculty.washington.edu/chudler/plast.html. So what does that mean? It means that we are finding that this drug very well could be interfering with brain maturation and plasticity, an unequivocal bad thing.

Very short, down and dirty, as we grow the brain is programmed to change shape, neurons are supposed to grow and die off; this drug (and perhaps others) could be inhibiting this process causing downstream deleterious effects. These effects have not been studied for long term usage. We simply do not know how it works, what the long term effects are, or what the dangers may be giving this drug to children as most studies are done on adults, not on children. With that said, let's move on to some of the other popular treatments.

Stimulants are also a very popular treatment for ADD/HD. "All stimulants work by increasing dopamine levels in the brain—dopamine is a brain chemical (or neurotransmitter) associated with pleasure, movement, and attention. The therapeutic effect of stimulants is achieved by slow and steady increases of dopamine, which are similar to the natural production of the chemical by the brain. The doses prescribed by physicians start low and increase gradually until a therapeutic effect is reached. However, when taken in doses and routes other than those prescribed, stimulants can increase brain dopamine in a rapid and highly amplified manner—as do most other drugs of abuse—disrupting normal communication between brain cells, producing euphoria, and increasing the risk of addiction. "according to NIDA a part of NIH.

Again, a part of the dopamine circuitry.

Strattera (Atomoxitine) is FDA approved for the treatment of ADD/HD. Atomoxitine was originally produced as an antidepressant, when it was proven to not be effective for that, it was used for treating ADD.[3] It is the only approved treatment for ADD/HD that is not a stimulant, and therefore less prone to abuse, according to the FDA.

In 2005 the FDA saw the necessity to release this "Public Health Advisory" http://www.fda.gov/NewsEvents/Newsroom/PressAnnouncements/2005/ucm108493.htm about the dangers of suicidal ideation while in treatment for ADD/HD, and has since been awarded a "black box" warning. "A black box warning is a warning that is seen on the package insert for prescription drugs that may cause serious adverse effects. A black border usually surrounds the text of the warning. It is also called a black label warning or boxed warning. "A black box warning indicates that medical studies show that the drug carries a considerable risk of serious or even life threatening adverse effects. The U.S. Food and Drug Administration may ask pharmaceutical companies to place a black box warning on the labeling of a prescription drug, or in literature describing it. It is the strongest warning that the FDA requires."[4] Let that sink in for a minute…hundreds of thousands of prescriptions have been written for this drug for children 6 and up…

Strattera is a Norepinephrine selective reuptake inhibitor. What that means is that when Norepinephrine is released into the neuronal synapse, it is not treated as the body would naturally treat it and be reabsorbed or broken down by enzymes. It is allowed to stay in the synaptic cleft and "cycle" causing the receptors to "uptake" it over and over.

- Norepinephrine is a hormone AND a neurotransmitter. As it breaks down (is metabolized) in the body it breaks into useful parts: Normetanephrine (via the enzyme catechol-O-methyl transferase, COMT)

- 3,4-Dihydroxymandelic acid (via monoamine oxidase, MAO)

- Vanillylmandelic acid (3-Methoxy-4-hydroxymandelic acid), also referred to as vanilmandelate or VMA (via MAO)

- 3-Methoxy-4-hydroxyphenylethylene glycol, "MHPG" or "MOPEG" (via MAO)

- Epinephrine (via PNMT)[15]

(More information can be found here: http://en.wikipedia.org/wiki/Norepinephrine)

Ok, so, if there is a bunch of Norepinephrine in the brain that is not being metabolized in a "natural" way, there is imbalance of some sort that have yet to be discovered, hence the side effects.

I now have a headache and I want to cry. I had some nebulous feeling that something was wrong, now I am convinced. Next time we are going to tackle off-labeling of drugs for ADD/HD. WARNING: Prepare to be PISSED!

References:

1. http://www.mclean.harvard.edu/news/press/current.php?id=65

2. http://www.nih.gov/news/health/feb2009/nida-02.htm

3. http://en.wikipedia.org/wiki/Strattera

4. http://definitions.uslegal.com/b/black-box-warning%20/

5. http://www.nida.nih.gov/infofacts/ADHD.html

The ADHD Scam and the Mass Drugging of School Children (excerpts)[7]

Today I am bringing you news from the world of ADHD, because scientists claim they have found a difference in the brains of children with ADHD

---

7 http://www.naturalnews.com/023334_child_children_brain.html#ixzz1EtNWtvQP

versus "normal" children. The brains of these children who have been diagnosed with ADHD were scanned with an MRI machine. They compared 40,000 different points in their brains looking for signs of thickness in the brain tissue.

They discovered that the brains of children diagnosed with ADHD were a little behind schedule in growing. Yes, you heard that right. They said they are about three years behind the brains of other children. Everything else was normal. They said if they wait three years those children will catch up and turn out just fine.

Now who is "they?" Dr. Phillip Shaw from the National Institute of Health, which is probably the National Institute of Mental Health -- they are the ones who did this research and this research has been making the rounds in mainstream media. You hear stories about it all over the radio. I heard one on national public radio today.

The Drugs Don't Work

It was a team of American scientists researching what is called the "Multi-Modal Treatment Study of Children with ADHD -- MTA for short. They found that the drugs are useless over long-term. The drugs used to treat ADHD such as Ritalin and Concerta are useless. They have no benefits whatsoever after three years and even though they may show some short-term benefits depending on who is watching, and depending on their judgment of the child's behavior, the truth is there is no long-term benefit whatsoever. But here's the most important part.

They found that these drugs stunt the growth of children. "They were not growing as much as other children in terms of both their height and their weight," said the report's co-author, Prof. William Pelham from the University of Buffalo. "I think we exaggerated the beneficial impact of medication in the first study," he added in reference to a study they did a few years ago where they declared that these drugs were helping children.

"We had thought that children medicated longer would have better outcomes. That did not happen to be the case. The children had a substantial decrease in their growth rate," he continued. The second point was that there were no benefits to children taking these drugs whatsoever.

What they did not say in the results of this study is that the same drugs also stunt the growth of the children's brains. Now this is my assessment of the situation, having studied this issue for several years and knowing that this drug is stunting the development of the children. It is very reasonable to conclude that it also stunts the growth of their brains and guess what? This new study actually proves it, because these MRI brain scans of children's brains that found that these brains were three years behind schedule in development.

80% of the children who were looked at with those MRI scans were on ADHD medications. That's right. All that study did was prove that medication stunts the growth of children's brains. Amazing is it not?

Drugging the Children in America: 84% of ADHD Kids Put on Medication[8]

According to a new survey by Consumer Reports, 84 percent of children diagnosed with attention deficit hyperactivity disorder (ADHD) are treated with drugs at some point.

Researchers from the magazine interviewed 934 parents whose children (under age 18) had been diagnosed with the disorder, asking them questions including which treatments they had used and how effective each of them had been. The survey was conducted online in July and August 2009.

Eighty-four percent children had taken drugs for the condition at some point. More than 50 percent had taken two or more different drugs in the past three years alone. The average age of children receiving drugs was 13; older children were more likely to take drugs than younger ones.

The two classes of ADHD drugs include stimulants, such as Ritalin, and non-stimulants, including atomoxetine (Strattera) and antidepressants. The stimulants include the amphetamines, such as Adderall, and the methylphenidates, such as Ritalin.

---

8 adhd news and articles - http://www.naturalnews.com/adhd.html#ixzz1EqgDX2K0

"We asked parents to rate how helpful each medication was in the following areas: academic performance, behavior at school, behavior at home, self-esteem, and social relationships," the authors wrote. "Both amphetamines and methylphenidates were equally likely to be helpful in all areas with the exception of behavior at school, where amphetamines were rated as slightly more helpful."

Among parents whose children had taken drugs, 67 percent said that the medication had helped "a lot." Thirty-five percent said that the drugs were most helpful at improving behavior at school and academic performance, 26 percent said the drugs had helped their child's social relationships, and 18 percent said they improved their child's self-esteem.

Even though the rate of psychiatric drug use was so high, only 22 percent of children were being seen by a psychiatrist; in contrast, 65 percent were receiving treatment from a pediatrician. Non-medical treatment providers included psychologists and learning-disability specialists.

Yet despite the high use of the drugs, parents did not appear to be comfortable relying on them. Only 52 percent of parents said that if they could go back and start over, they would give their children drugs, while 44 percent said they wished there were a non-pharmaceutical way to help their child.

Part of this dissatisfaction may have come from side effects, which were experienced by 84 percent of children who took drugs. The most commonly reported adverse effects were digestive upset, decreased appetite, irritability, trouble sleeping and weight loss.

The high rate of side effects suggests that doctors might not be adjusting dosage properly to account for different patients, said neurologist Orly Avitzur, a medical adviser to Consumer Reports.

"It's not like you can just give the child a pill and you're finished," she explains. "There's a lot more to it in terms of management."

According to Patrick Tolan of the University of Virginia, drugs are simply not capable of correcting all ADHD-related problems.

"With medication, the child isn't so distracted, and that makes it easier to learn," he said. "But it's not going to teach the child problem-solving skills or give him the ability to stop and think things through like other kids do."

Indeed, the excessive use of medication to regulate children's behavior is one of the primary criticisms leveled at the ADHD diagnosis.

"If the forcing of the ADHD diagnosis and drugs can be justified, then why not do it for every other condition? After all, it is for the good of the child, right?" writes Fred A. Baughman, Jr. and Craig Hovey in The ADHD Fraud.

"The problem, of course, is that ... anything that disturbs adults in authority can be classified as a disease and parents threatened with the loss of their children if they don't go along with 'treatment.' Do any of us want this to happen, to witness childhood itself held hostage by drug pushers?"[9]

(Dr. Kevin says...)

I want to comment here on some of these findings. In my years of working with both children and adults I do consistently find that the medications have been listed as helpful for a number of reasons. However, key points are not being looked at in the equation. In speaking with children I have often found that their willingness to be on the medication has more to do with pleasing other people, getting into less trouble, not feeling isolated. They didn't like how it made them feel and complained about the other side effects. It was a lesser of two evils choice. I have thought more than once that it provides the same benefit that alcohol or certain other mind-altering drugs do, it helps you fit in.

As far as for better academic results, perhaps the better question is are they living up to their potential or do the drugs allow them to perform down at "average" students potential? Do they look better because they are better able to deal with mediocre educational requirements? As pointed out above, medication does not teach thinking or thinking things through. But can we say that public education does those things for any of our children? How much of that should be being taught or reinforced in a stable consistent family unit? Are parents being asked to teach and role model skill sets that they do not have? In the 21st century will it be more important for these children to think outside the box instead of in it? Will problem solving skills and self-awareness be more important than memorization and the robotic following of instruction? Do we need to be developing more leaders and fewer followers? Do we need more challenging and engaged and less apathetic, dependent and medicated children and adults? Sure there is a pill for everything but at what cost?

---

9 *Sources for this story include:*http://www.msnbc.msn.com/id/3831590... http://www.webmd.com/add-adhd/news/....

The Business of ADHD[10]

Psychiatrists convened in sunny Honolulu for the 164th Annual Meeting of the American Psychiatric Association (APA) last week, discussing, among other things, moving forward with plans to make the diagnostic criteria for ADHD less stringent: proposed changes include reducing the number of required symptoms from 6 to 4, for adults and teens, and increasing the age-of-onset criteria from 7 to 12.

Russell Barkley, Ph.D., and Joseph Biederman, M.D., have written about abandoning or generously broadening age-of-onset criteria, arguing that the current, precise age-of-onset criteria poses "unwarranted practical problems for the study of older adolescents and adults." These two men are considered ADHD experts and contributed to the American Academy of Child and Adolescent Psychiatry (AACAP) Practice Parameters for ADHD, which serve as guidelines by which most child psychiatrists practice.

According to a story from the *New York Times*, Joseph Biederman did not tell university officials about more than a million dollars received from drugmakers from 2000 to 2007, and he promised Johnson & Johnson research results that would benefit the drug company. On the list of AACAP Conflicts of Interests for Practice Parameters not listed in the Practice Parameters, Russell Barkley receives or has received research support, acted as a consultant and/or served on a speaker's bureau for Eli Lilly and Company and Shire Pharmaceuticals Group.

Shire Pharmaceuticals Group has a substantial focus on ADHD meds, and they have been pulling out all the stops to try and turn a profit in the face of competition from generic drugs.

Earlier this month, *Reuter's Health* described how drugmakers, including Shire, have raised prices to make up for lack of new products and loss of patent protection.

"Prices were just shoved up every year to make more money and meet earnings, to be blunt," Shire (SHP.L) Chief Executive Angus Russell said.

Shire's CEO also indicated that the FDA is supporting their plan to study the use of their ADHD drug, Vyvanse, for use in depression and schizophrenia,

---

10 http://www.sfgate.com/cgi-bin/blogs/wchung/detail?entry_id=89494

hoping for billions of dollars in extra sales through expansion of potential indications. Amphetamines for schizophrenia? Hmmmm.....

Jim Edwards of BNET wrote about Shire increasing the price of one of their own ADHD drugs, Adderall XR, to encourage users to switch to their branded, cheaper and newer ADHD drug, Vyvanse, leading to increased sales.

Shire somehow sold more ADHD drugs during a recent, national shortage of ADHD medications - their sales of Adderall XR increased 21 percent in the first quarter of 2011 - a time when many of the patients in San Francisco's public mental health system were unable to receive their regular ADHD medications.

BNET posted excerpts of separate lawsuits filed by Impax and Teva, manufacturers of generic forms of Adderall XR. They claim that Shire did not honor their contracts and hoarded product for themselves during this recent shortage. In the *Wall Street Journal*, the associate director of FDA's drug shortages program reported that this national ADHD drug shortage mostly affected generic forms of ADHD meds. Coincidence?

Other ways of getting around stagnant drug development and generic competition include taking an old drug or active ingredient, and changing the delivery system or duration of action and presenting it as a new, patent-protected product. Here are a few examples that have been associated with Shire:

- Vyvanse: Also known as lisdexamfetamine, Vyvanse is a prodrug of dextroamphetamine. Dextroamphetamine has been used since 1937 to treat hyperactivity in children, so it is hardly new. Vyvanse was marketed as having lower abuse potential - specifically, preventing abuse from snorting, since the prodrug requires digestion to release the active form. In my clinical experience, most abuse of stimulants is due to people taking it without a prescription or shaping their symptoms to get a prescription, and a prodrug likely does little to curb college students from seeking stimulants to study for exams.

- Daytrana: The transdermal methylphenidate (methylphenidate is the active ingredient in Ritalin) patch is worn on the skin and was developed as a way of bypassing the digestive tract, and my experience prescribing this drug was met with equivocal reports from patients and families. I guess there is a reason I can't remember anyone saying it worked - Shire gave up on the ADHD patch after 9 product recalls and a federal probe.

- Intuniv: An extended release form of guanfacine, Intuniv is touted as a new, non-stimulant treatment for ADHD. But child psychiatrists have been using guanfacine in ADHD for years, and this 'extended-release' form has a half-life of about 18 hours, while generic guanfacine has a half-life of about 17 hours - not a robust difference, in my opinion.

I liken these approaches to gimmicks utilized in the mass-produced, beer market: color changing <u>labels</u> to let you know if your beer is cold, <u>wide-mouth</u> beer cans, or <u>vortex</u> bottles. Do any of these 'innovations' really change the fact that you're drinking cheap beer?

As the DSM-V looms closer to becoming a reality, I can't help but think of words from the man who chaired the committee for the DSM-IV. Allen Frances, M.D., <u>wrote</u> in the in the *LA Times*:

As chairman of the task force that created the current Diagnostic and Statistical Manual of Mental Disorders (DSM-IV), which came out in 1994, I learned from painful experience how small changes in the definition of mental disorders can create huge, unintended consequences.

Our panel tried hard to be conservative and careful but inadvertently contributed to three false 'epidemics' - attention deficit disorder, autism and childhood bipolar disorder. Clearly, our net was cast too wide and captured many 'patients' who might have been far better off never entering the mental health system.

The DSM-IV was and the DSM-V will be published by the APA. The same APA that, in 2010, rejected internal recommendations - led by an APA past-president - to regulate or curtail individual psychiatrists' relationships with the pharmaceutical industry.

Loosening the diagnostic criteria for ADHD, as proposed, will no doubt lead to more people being diagnosed and, inevitably, taking more ADHD drugs. I like to think that the APA and their doctors pushing for the changes are motivated by helping patients and not drug company profits.

After all, if anyone can identify and address unconscious conflicts or psychologically-defended, aggressive drives, it's a psychiatrist, right?

CHAPTER 9

SUPPORTING CAST

As ADD, THEN ADHD and now as I like to refer to it ADD/HD hit the public consciousness as a set of diagnoses, the majority of people jumped on the "how can we cure, fix, heal or eliminate this disability which is causing so much heartache, strife and disruptiveness in schools and homes" bandwagon. There were a handful of us that saw it in a different way. We had some that wanted to see it as bad parenting, others as a problematic school system, another blamed computers, video games and TV for the onset of ADD/HD, and still another was a proponent of diet, environmental toxicities, and the dramatic increase in vaccinations.

At the same time as all of this, there was the beginning of what became known as the Indigo Child movement which I was extremely vocal about because in their earliest work they tried to separate the ADD issue and ADD child out from Indigo Child. The Indigo Child was all shiny and new and a new child on the planet and the ADD child was, oh well, ADD. At that time I accused that approach as being self serving, taking the children who were different but less hassle and calling them Indigo and taking "my ADD kids" and leaving them behind trapped in the Ritalin noose. And though I was just as vocal about the injustices of rushing to the drug solution as to separating out the Indigo child from the ill-behaved, out of control ADD child, I was always closer to the Indigo view except as with so much of what I have done I took it several steps further and with some different perspectives.

Each group took its perspective and applied its set of tools and skill sets to the problem. Henceforth, we now have a variety of drugs, systems, herbs, supplements, and approaches and thought processes trying to solve the problems associated with ADD/HD which oftentimes are problems whose causes have not been fully defined.

I have been consistent with a few facts from my perspective of ADD/HD. First, it is an evolutionary process; second, it is not a disability but a diffability; third, the majority of issues we experience with the individual who is gifted with ADD/HD has more to do with them functioning in a non-ADD/HD world; fourth, environmental factors, such as diet, lighting, chemical and metal toxicity within the body, as well as societal issues, ill fitting educational systems and popular parenting and adult support systems exacerbate all the gifts into curses.

In this section are not miracle cures or fixes, but options that either help with the side effects of being in a highly toxic and ill-fitting world or tools and skills that help the child better fit in.

Some would say that all the work that I do falls into the category of alternative. And if one were to define alternative as alternative to drug based therapy, then I would agree. In this chapter however, I will be sharing some of the alternatives that I have had personal experience with as well as treatments which I have come across.

So what I will be presenting to you here are methods which I would recommend checking out. Which does not mean that I recommend doing them, but rather checking them out for yourself. One of my problems with alternatives is that I use them on a case by case basis depending on what I pick up from the individual with whom I am working. And they can vary greatly from individual to individual.

There are so many systems, supplements, and developmental tools out there such that besides the ones I know of or have worked with that I could spend the next several years trying them all out. In my first book I immediately eliminated them for one of two reasons. Either they claimed to "cure" a list of issues as long as my arm or they approached ADD/HD as something undesirable that it would help get rid of. Both of these I felt immediately discredit it from inclusion into this book. Now I see it differently. Although miracle cures still grate on my nerves and I still refuse to see ADD/HD as something that needs to be cured or even can be cured, it doesn't mean that some of the systems, supplements and such that fall into that category might not have some validity as a supporting cast member in a protocol which helps ADD/HD better manage their gifts.

Another point to consider that some recommendations that I make have nothing to do with the ADD/HD impact itself. Some factors, such as sensitivities to diet and environment, at first glance are seen as negative when actually they are part of the gift. They are part of the gift because they force us to be more aware and make better choices when it comes to what we eat and what is present in the environment around us.

As we examine the following potential solutions keep in mind that they offer help from a number of different perspectives and through dealing with different aspects of the negative impacts that the ADD/HD has on your child. A comprehensive well planned and consistently implemented approach will always work best over time. No magic pills, wands or epiphanies will miraculously make your child "normal". Which is a very good thing.

Chiropractic

Chiropractic focuses on the disorders of the musculoskeletal system and the nervous system, and the effects of these disorders on general health. Chiropractic is most often utilized to treat neuromusculoskeletal complaints, including but not limited to back pain, neck pain, pain in the joints of the arms or legs, and headaches.

Chiropractic physicians practice a drug-free, hands-on approach to health care that includes patient examination, diagnosis and treatment. Through their training, they have broad diagnostic skills and may also recommend therapeutic and rehabilitative exercises, as well as to provide nutritional, dietary and lifestyle counseling. Here is what the American Chiropractic Association has to say about the work they are doing with ADD/HD individuals.

Although currently no studies comparing chiropractic neurological and medical treatment for ADHD are available, chiropractic neurologists are compiling the data. "We test children before they start the treatment and then every three months," says Dr. Melillo. "Within the first three months, the children get a two-grade-level increase on average—which is pretty dramatic. With children on medications, the improvement in academic performance is short term and lasts only as long as they take the medication. Our programs change the brain function and the improvement doesn't go away."[11]

Personally I use and recommend this modality as part of a holistic way to help support the gifts of ADD/HD.

Homeopathy

Homeopathy is a holistic approach to healing which considers the physical, emotional, and mental symptoms or patterns of the individual. The body can be brought back into balance and health by stimulating its natural defense mechanism through the use of "remedies". Remedies are mostly derived from animal, plant, or mineral sources. They are ingested in pellet, tablet or liquid form and come in various potencies or strengths. Remedies can be used both preventively to strengthen the immune system or when acute or chronic symptoms are manifesting. Homeopathic remedies are nontoxic and do not cause side effects because they are very diluted. They work on a vibrational level.

When considering how to manage the "symptoms" of ADD/HD homeopathically a consultation with a homeopathic practitioner is recommended. This consultation is much more in depth than those of allopathic practitioners, and can take between 1-2 hours to complete. The homeopath will "take the case" or gather as much information as possible about the emotional, mental and physical symptoms by asking questions and observing the client. This information is compared to the symptoms associated with various remedies. Each remedy has a "picture" of symptoms, which the remedy has been known to cure or positively affect. When a match is made between a remedies picture of symptoms and those symptoms manifesting in the client, this single remedy is given to the client. This is known as "the law of similars" or like cures like. The client is then monitored for his/her response to the remedy.

---

11 (http://www.acatoday.org/content_css.cfm?CID=60)

Flower Essences

A flower essence is the vibrational (energy) pattern of a flower which brings balance to a person on all levels: physical, emotional, mental and spiritual. Basically, placing the flower's petals in a bowl of clean water and setting them in the sun for about 3 hours makes a flower essence. This releases the specific healing and balancing pattern of the flower into the water in a very condensed form. The petals are removed and this tincture is diluted and preserved with brandy. The essence is taken orally a few drops at a time.

Flower essence helps to heal, balance and strengthen our electrical energy system. Our electrical system can become short-circuited or shut down as we go through life. Unless this is corrected, our bodies can be cut off from the electrical life force energy they need to be healthy, and may experience pain, illness or disease. Overload of the electrical system can also occur which may cause hyperactivity and twitching. Essences are able to reconnect and rebalance the circuitry in the body. Since people with ADD/HD seem to have very well developed nervous systems, are very sensitive to energy, and tend to be energetically on overload, they can greatly benefit from using flower essences.

Flower essences also address the mental and emotional patterns in our etheric bodies which contain our destructive mental, spiritual and emotional illusions or blocks. These blocks vibrate at a slow rate. Because the essences vibrate at a higher rate, they help to facilitate the release of these blocks. When our blocks are released, we can open more to receive the healing energies of Spirit.

Flower essences are extremely safe. If a person does ingest an essence his/her body does not need, then there is no pattern to be released and therefore there is no effect. There are absolutely no side effects at all. They are extremely powerful, yet extremely gentle.

Biofeedback/ Neurofeedback

Biofeedback is a process in which information on how a person's body and brain are working is amplified and shown back to that person. For example, various devices are used to measure muscle tension and body temperature which help people to learn to regulate their blood pressure, temperature and other physical and mental functions that are not usually consciously controlled. Biofeedback is used to treat stress-related conditions like migraine headaches and chronic pain.

Neurofeedback is a form of biofeedback also referred to as an EEG biofeedback. It uses an electroencephalograph to train a person to alter his/her brain wave patterns. Electrodes are placed on the scalp which sense brain wave activity. There is no pain associated with this and no electricity goes into the brain. The brain wave information is sent into a computer which translates them into pictures. The person is able to change his/her brain waves by watching how these brain waves affect the pictures on the computer. Computer games for children are now available which require the use of mind power alone to play. The child learns to affect the game by increasing or decreasing certain brain waves. In effect, neurofeedback retrains the brain to produce the desired brain waves.

Brain Waves:

The 4 kinds of brain waves are:

1. Delta: .5 - 4 cycles/ second or .5 - 4 hertz (HZ) – Deep sleep

2. Theta: 4 - 8 HZ – Dreamy, deep meditation

3. Alpha: 8 - 12 HZ – Calm, mentally unfocused, relaxed wakefulness

4. Beta: 12 - 15 HZ – Alert concentration, normal waking state up to 35 HZ – High beta, excited, anxious

Studies have shown that boys and girls with ADD/HD produce more theta brain waves and less beta waves than children without ADD/HD.[12] Neurofeedback teaches children and adults to control their minds so that they can increase the amount of beta waves they produce, while decreasing the theta waves. Therefore, they are more able to focus their attention and concentration.

Sessions:

It takes about 40-80 sessions (40-60 minutes per session), or some sources[13] say 20-40 sessions to produce lasting EEG and clinical changes. Follow-up

---

12 Article: "Attention Deficit Hyperactivity, Disorder: Neurological Basis and Treatment Alternatives". http://www.snrjnt.org/

13 Eeg Spectrum International™ - www.eegspectrum.com

assessments should be done at about 1 month, 6 months and 1 year after the treatment is complete.[14]

Results:

Follow-up studies on children who have received Neurofeedback training have shown significant increases in academic and behavior scores. Some children have advanced up to 2.5 years in grade level achievement and increased I.Q. scores as much as 15 points.[15]

Ingestions: Supportive and Otherwise

We have all heard some variation of, "You are what you eat". In this upcoming section we are going to break it down into three categories: Heroes (what and how to eat), Sidekicks (helpful supplementation) and Villains (known troublemakers). Some of this is diet but it also encompasses supplements and herbs.

Heroes and Villains

Part of the evolutionary shift that has been made within these individuals is that they are more nutrient based than caloric based. The shift in overall diet for the last fifty years has moved to a diet which has less naturally occurring vitamins, minerals and nutrients, with significant parts of that diet containing little or none at all. The body does not respond the same way to foods which have been highly processed and prepared even if the foods have been enriched with those missing vitamins and minerals. Also, because of farming techniques and the change to mass production, the foods coming out of the actual ground itself have fewer nutrients in them. So these children's bodies now search for nutrients instead of calories.

One of the reasons they may overeat has nothing to do with hunger but the body trying to find enough of the building blocks needed from food so that

---

14 ADHD: Neurological Basis and Treatment Alternatives". www.snr-jnt.org/

15 Article by John Robbins, "Wired for Miracles". March/April, 1996 - www. eggspectrum.com/

they can function at the high level that they are capable of in a productive and successful way. When I have dramatically increased the nutrients which the child is receiving, their desire for junk food goes down and their ability to function within acceptable limits goes up. Now again, I caution here that while diet is an integral part of helping your ADD/HD child (or adult) to live up to their potential, diet alone won't do it, but must be part of the process.

Keep some of the following facts in mind. The average diet today is higher in calories, fats, sodium and sugar then ever. According to Eco Salon[16] our current percentage of overweight and obese children is 33% and the percentage of fast food meals that make up our diet is 55%.

A diet rich in whole foods, organic, lightly cooked or raw foods is always a good bet. Also a diet that is more alkaline in nature is helpful. The average western diet is extremely acidic. Besides the fact that an overly acidic body will have more health issues, it can also stimulate more irritation and hyperactivity. An over acidic child is a child that is more likely to grumpy, get sick and be more restless.

Go for natural, unprocessed, and highly nutritious foods, eating smaller meals with plenty of grazing in between. If the child eats only highly nutritious food, he will have smoother energy with fewer peaks and physically based meltdowns. The child's systems need to process the food without becoming overwhelmed by too many calories or irritated by eating chemically altered food which I call "fake" food. The ADD/HD individual, on the whole, seems to have less tolerance for and is more impacted by large meals and "fake" food than the average person, a reality that plays out in bad behaviors.

Because these individuals are more nutrient-based than caloric-based, you have to be careful they do not develop a tendency to overeat the wrong kinds of food. When they eat "fake" food, their bodies sense that they need more nutrients, and even though they are physically full, they still crave food. Because of the built-in addictive nature of many of these kinds of foods, their desire becomes not only for actual nutrients but also for chemically altered, "fake" foods. This creates a dangerous cycle, which can contribute to meltdowns and focus issues and can lead to anger and other negative play-outs.

I have often times found sensitivities to drugs, overly/heavily processed foods, caffeine, dairy, and sometimes even wheat, which is not to say that every-

16 (www.ecosalon.com)

one who is impacted with the ADD/HD will have any or all these sensitivities, but they are things to watch out for. Eliminating things with food coloring and dyes is highly recommended. As well as eliminating foods heavily processed with lots of chemicals tends to make a big difference.

Sidekicks

Spirulina is a super food rich in vitamins, chelated minerals, and trace minerals. It's a concentrated source of beta-carotene and is one of the highest sources of chlorophyll. It consists of up to 69% of balanced high quality vegetable protein, containing all eight essential amino acids which the body uses to create complete proteins. I personally like it in a form called *Life Source* where it is available in either capsules or a powder form and is mixed in with all the other high nutritional value which contains not only Spirulina, but a whole host of super greens which gives it a more well rounded punch of nutrients than Spirulina alone. Here is a partial list of what Life Source[17] has in it:

Spirulina, Chlorella, Chlorophyll, Alfalfa, Wheat Grass, Barley Juice, Carrot Powder, Flax Seed (an excellent source of Omega 3, 6, 8)

Because it comes in powder and capsules it can be used in a smoothie format or just as capsules. Within a smoothie or separately, the addition of L-tyrosine and some additional Omega-3's, many have found helpful. Consider doing this twice a day, before going to school and as part of the after school snack. I am a big supporter of smoothies created with those extra supporting nutrients, as well as fresh fruits, and natural flavorings. These can have a powerful stabilizing boost that helps your child have greater ability to focus and stay more emotionally stable.

Rare and essential fatty acids, such as Omega 3's, are also contained in blue-green algae. It is a blood purifier and a powerful antiseptic which seeks out and eliminates toxins (free radicals) in the body. Essential fatty acids (EFA'S) are necessary for health. All of them are made by the body except for Omega-3 and Omega 6. These fats are especially needed for the healthy functioning of

---

17 Additional information about *Life Source* can be found on my website www. managingthegift.com

the heart, brain and cell membranes. In addition to the focus on EFA's, I also found that an herbal combination of L-Tyrosine and B Complex helped many of my clients. See a qualified herbal health practitioner or do the research, then decide if you would like to try it.

Therapeutic Magnets

Individuals in tune with the use of magnets as a healing tool began magnetic therapies to help initially with the side effects of the ADD/HD individual living in a non-ADD/HD world. Dr Daniel T. Moore in his paper on ADHD treatment Classification was more vocal in his support for therapeutic magnets as well as some other things we have discussed here. He said:

> Environmental controls include methods to adjust the child's environment to relieve ADHD symptoms. These techniques include diet, detoxing the body, and having a Nikken Wellness Home. The Feingold diet and the elimination diet are examples of an environmental control. Nikken, a different environmental approach, recommends that children are raised within a Wellness Home (sleep system, air filter, water filter, nutritional products) to help children overcome their ADHD symptoms. Dr. Melaney Caldwell, a pediatrician, believes that a Nikken Wellness Home is more effective than medication for ADHD symptoms.[18]

I believe that the correct magnets applied in the correct format can help with some of those issues that exacerbate ADD/HD traits to a high alert problem level. I also feel that it creates an internal supporting system through deeper and better sleep as well as strengthening internal support factors to better deal with some of the ADD/HD impacts that can get in the way of day to day living.

---

18 ADHD Treatment Classifications by Daniel T. Moore, Ph.D. (www. yourfamilyclinic.com/adhd/adhdtreatmentmethods.html)

Full Spectrum Lighting

For some children with ADD/HD, the pulsing pattern that exists within florescent lighting can have a significantly noticeable and disruptive effect which affects their mood and focus ability. Here is some research that was done by Dr. William Campbell Douglass in his book, _Into the Light_,

> _The cameras recording the activity of the children exposed to full-spectrum light recorded a marked decrease in hyperactivity among the children, with a definite calming effect and an increase in their attention span compared to those exposed to the "cool white," non-full-spectrum lights._ _In particular, several extremely hyperactive children with "confirmed learning disabilities" calmed down completely and rapidly overcame their "learning disabilities" under the full-spectrum light._ _The overall academic achievement level of those exposed to full-spectrum light was superior to those under the deficient lights, and, perhaps the most incredible finding of all, dentists found that those children exposed to full-spectrum light developed only one-third the number of cavities as those under the "cool white" fluorescent lighting._[19]

Cleansing and Detoxing

Because of the sensitive nature of the physical bodies of the ADD/HD child, the build up of chemicals and metals within these children definitely adds to the kinds of behaviors, which lead to the perceived need that the only way to manage them is through medicating them. I have included this research study done by Roger D. Masters   Department of Government, Dartmouth College Foundation for Neuroscience and Society to illuminate this concern.

> _Silicofluoride (SiF) treated water can increase the transport of heavy metals across the gut-blood and blood-brain barriers, increasing rates of toxic uptake and behavioral dysfunction. Minorities are especially at risk. The brain is the most sensitive chemical organ in the body. In contemporary society, these effects take on a different_

---

19 Dr. William Campbell Douglass, Into the Light, page 189.

character. Environmental pollution and dangerous water treatment procedures are human activities whose results are both economically costly and morally unjust. Innocent children should not be poisoned by public water supplies.

Summary: Heavy metals compromise normal brain development and neurotransmitter function, leading to long-term deficits in learning and social behavior. At the individual level, earlier studies revealed that hyperactive children and criminal offenders have significantly elevated levels of lead, manganese, or cadmium compared to controls; high blood lead at age seven predicts juvenile delinquency and adult crime. At the environmental level, our research has found that environmental factors associated with toxicity are correlated with higher rates of anti-social behavior. For the period 1977 to 1997, levels of violent crime and teenage homicide were significantly correlated with the probability of prenatal and infant exposure to leaded gasoline years earlier. Across all U.S. counties for both 1985 and 1991, industrial releases of heavy metals were -- controlling for over 20 socio-economic and demographic factors -- also a risk-factor for higher rates of crime. Surveys of children's blood lead in Massachusetts, New York, and other states as well as NHANES III and an NIJ study of 24 cities point to another environmental factor: where silicofluorides are used as water treatment agents, risk-ratios for blood lead over 10μg/dL are from 1.25 to 2.5, with significant interactions between the silicofluorides and other factors associated with lead uptake. Communities using silicofluorides also report higher rates of learning disabilities, ADHD, violent crime, and criminals who were using cocaine at the time of arrest.[20]

Energy Work

Visualizations, identifying and working with energy, meditation and shielding helps. I also teach my clients breathing and centering exercises. These are all tools I can work with my clients to do on their own which help

---

20 *Poisoning the Well: Neurotoxic Metals, Water Treatment, and Human Behavior* Roger D. Masters. Research conducted with Myron J. Coplan (Intellequity, Natick, MA) and Brian Hone under grants from the Office of Criminal Enforcement, Forensics and Training, Environmental Protection Agency, the Earhart Foundation, and the Rockefeller Center for the Social Sciences, Dartmouth College.

manage the times of excess energy, or mental overload. Some of my clients have benefited from practicing a martial art, Tai Chi, or yoga. Also dance classes, sports, working with their hands are all things which can help as well as being used as ways to make learning more kinesthetic, in approach, which is helpful.

If you are looking for shielding meditations, I recommend the book *Invisible Armor: Protecting Your Personal Energy*, or the CD *Creating Your Invisible Armor* both of which are by Thomas Hensel. In addition, my Managing The Gift Daily Practices CD has both AM and PM meditations which combines shielding with an emotional coffee break component. In particular, the AM meditation helps to organize and set the direction of the day which can facilitate a smoother experience.

To Keep In Mind

There are many alternatives out there; I have just begun to scratch the surface. The important is to be clear on what you are trying to accomplish, avoid miracle drugs, get referrals when possible and take the responsibility of doing your own legwork. Not all supplements, herbs, aromatherapies, magnets, full spectrum lights, etcetera are the same. If you want to make sure that you that you get the right one or the highest quality then please feel free go to my website: www.*managingthegift.com* and you will find a complete list of the resources I recommend. Here is an example of why I have created the section on my website, aromatherapies, you can go to your local box store and buy an aromatherapy scented candle or oil and diffuser or pay a higher cost and get a true essential oil. The difference is what you are most likely buying is a scent from of petroleum oil, which smells good but does very little in helping. In fact burning it is paramount to sniffing car fumes, nice smelling car fumes, but car fumes, which may actually trigger other negative play-outs and not help. So then what happens is that you actually have more problems then you started with and you tell yourself and everyone else that aromatherapies don't help.

Additional Resources:

- Dance Dance Revolution is a great game to develop attention skills in ADHD children.

- Brain Train (www.braintrain.com) makes computer software in the form of video games that improve ADHD symptoms.

- Most developmental learning programs (e.g, Pace Tutoring, DORE, SOI) will also affect attention abilities. According to Pace Tutoring (www.pacetutoring.com) research results, they are able to advance a child's attention skills by four years within a three month period. There are a wide variety of neuro-developmental exercises now available to treat ADHD symptoms. The advantage of these techniques is that once the neuro-developmental pathways are developed or learning has taken place, the results are permanent (unless exposed to additional toxins or injury).

CHAPTER 10

IN CONCLUSION

HOW WE SEE something determines how we treat it. As long as we see ADD/HD as a disability that is best treated with medication then we will treat it that way. By doing this we also take children who do have challenges and set them up with a label, which does not serve them, and does not help them.

Medications may help them on a temporary basis, to fit in, to adjust to situations such as problems with an educational system that does not know how to help these children to manage all their energy, brilliance & creativity without medication. With the introduction of medication, other issues and problems get both masked and get created.

Medication makes lots of people's life easier and sometimes the immediate relief overshadows the cost, both short term and long term. Sometimes it doesn't but when parents are faced with what comes across as the only solution, what are they to do? What choice so they have? But there are choices. Unfortunately, those choices get played down or discarded because either they cost too much in time and effort or too many changes have to be made.

There is also the fact that lots of money gets made and goes into the flow. Lots of money. Money which gets reinvested into advertising and support for the non-profits, people & politicians that support a "disabled and needs to be medicated" reality.

Am I saying medicine is always bad, and should never be used? No, I won't say that. Limited in special situations I am sure it is appropriate, as long as other things are in place so that it is a temporary fix only.

For over 150 years, we have been watching as humanity has been evolving to new heights, new depths and expanding at a rate, hitherto unheard of. These individuals, that we call ADD/HD have been the architects of those changes. Quantum physics tells us that we only take in a minute fraction of the stimuli that surrounds us. We have been taught that we only access about 10% of our brains capacity. We prove over and over again that we have the ability to far succeed where the generation before has brought us. As the world has become smaller, more connected and more interdependent upon itself, and expanded to a population that would have been considered unimaginable even a hundred years ago, we have been giving more and more power to institutions to keep the world and its populations functioning, flowing, and in order.

The trouble is that institutions reach a point where their true primary mission is not about serving the people they were created to serve but to protect the institution itself. Here in the 21st century the institutions of government, education, social services, and the institutions related to medicine all have a vested interest in protecting themselves and staying in power, as well as growing their power or increasing their profits. The job of a business is to stay in business and deliver profits to its stockholders. Both these entities have higher level commitments than to the long term wellness of the child.

Am I being an alarmist? Maybe, but how would things be seen differently, handled differently and be different if we didn't see those individuals as disabled, broken, if we worked harder to fix systems and institutions that are broken, and delved deeper into understanding the issues, creating the systems and taking the time necessary that these children need. We hear about that these children and we are told about how their brains are smaller in certain sections but what we are not told is that 80% of the children that the scans were done on were children who had already been on ADD/HD medication. We aren't told that there is evidence that given enough time - three years, that the ADD/HD brain differences that cause the most difficulty in adjusting in the world, without having to medicate. There is so much we are not told or are only partially told. What we are told are the parts that allow this to continue being diagnosed as a disability. We are told the part that supports a medicine-based approach. We are told the part that the people who are making millions of dollars every year want us to know.

When you see your child are they really disabled? If there is ANY question in your mind that says they are not, that maybe they need some extra help, or additional supports for a time or need to be handled differently than the "average" child, does than don't make them disabled, don't let the world make them disabled. Don't give them an excuse to be less than they are. Helping them discover all that they are and help them get there, without a label. I said in my first book that it is not a disability- it is a diff-ability, they simply learn and process differently. I stand by that. Does doing things differently really deserve a label and a life of being medicated, being less than who they are here to be?

In these times it often seems hard to find hope for the future. There seems to be a focus on everything from the death of the planet to the mass destruction of man at his own hands. Yet when I wish to find hope for that future I turn to "my kids", my ADD/HD kids that is. I don't care whether they are eight or eighty there is always something childlike about them that automatically makes me call them my kids. For when I see these kids, spend time with these kids, touch their passion, hear their brilliance and experience their creative genius, I find hope. And one of the reasons I fight so hard to not let the world drug 'em up and dumb 'em down is because though it might be easier, more convenient and certainly more profitable, it interferes with why they are here, which is to give us hope and to show us the next level of human potential.

Made in the USA
Middletown, DE
04 February 2021